THE STATE OF DESIRE

# The State of Desire

*Religion and Reproductive Politics
in the Promised Land*

Lea Taragin-Zeller

NEW YORK UNIVERSITY PRESS
*New York*

NEW YORK UNIVERSITY PRESS
New York
www.nyupress.org

© 2023 by New York University
All rights reserved

Please contact the Library of Congress for Cataloging-in-Publication data.
ISBN: 9781479817351 (hardback)
ISBN: 9781479817368 (paperback)
ISBN: 9781479817382 (library ebook)
ISBN: 9781479817375 (consumer ebook)

New York University Press books are printed on acid-free paper, and their binding materials are chosen for strength and durability. We strive to use environmentally responsible suppliers and materials to the greatest extent possible in publishing our books.

Manufactured in the United States of America

10 9 8 7 6 5 4 3 2 1

Also available as an ebook

## CONTENTS

| | |
|---|---|
| Introduction | 1 |
| 1. Cracks | 43 |
| 2. Repro-Theologies in the Promised Land | 64 |
| 3. Creating an Ethical Language | 89 |
| 4. Reorienting Decision-Making | 105 |
| 5. Ending | 122 |
| *Coda* | 139 |
| *Acknowledgments* | 149 |
| *Notes* | 153 |
| *Bibliography* | 165 |
| *Index* | 183 |
| *About the Author* | 191 |

# Introduction

What does it mean to be oriented?
—Sara Ahmed, *Queer Phenomenology:
Orientations, Objects, Others*

Shlomo was a young religious man, with shining brown eyes and a large smile surrounded by a bushy beard. At age thirty-one, with three children under the age of four, Shlomo told me he was "barely breathing." He had been married for almost six years, and the constant juggle of work, kids, and a mortgage for his family's home in Jerusalem was taking its toll. Shlomo felt that his life was falling apart.

When Shlomo was twenty-five, he was introduced to Miriam, who was one year younger than him and new to religious observance. Even though he came from a rabbinic family, and she came from a secular Jewish family with a big passion for music, they fell in love immediately. They got engaged after dating for two months and never touched before they got married three months later. They had also never discussed contraception.

As the wedding approached, Shlomo told me, he started worrying. "I suddenly realized she was going to get pregnant."[1] As the wedding drew closer, Shlomo became more and more anxious. At that point, right before their wedding, Shlomo was not allowed to meet Miriam face-to-face and did not want to have this type of conversation over the phone. He spoke to his rabbi, who explained that with so little time there was no use to start taking hormonal pills, and if Shlomo wanted to, he would need to purchase something "mechanical." "Condoms are not permissible, but maybe you could purchase a sponge," the rabbi suggested. Shlomo had no idea what the rabbi was talking about. He realized he must talk to Miriam. Shlomo smiles sheepishly when he tells me what happened next: "I called her on the day of our wedding and told her I was scared to have children. Miriam was so angry. Apparently, I had picked the worst timing ever. I called when she was with her friends, getting her makeup done. She was so upset. She said: 'I am going to kill you!'"

Shlomo paused and looked out the window. Miriam really wanted to get pregnant immediately. She had always said how much she could not wait to get married, immediately have a belly, and have a child before their first anniversary. This was the conventional order of events, and that is what she yearned for. Even though Miriam was eager to get pregnant, she realized how scared Shlomo was and agreed to begin using contraception on their wedding night.

But not for long. Miriam succeeded in calming Shlomo down, and they had a baby boy within a year of their marriage. They were both thrilled. After their son was born, they decided to try to prevent conception, but if Miriam would get pregnant, they would be OK with it. After a year she was pregnant again, and another boy was born. But this time, Shlomo said, it was harder. Life turned into chaos. Even though both Miriam and Shlomo grew up in Jerusalem, they moved north to join a small religious community, hoping rural life would prove less costly. "It was a typical situation of a low-income but highly spiritual community," Shlomo explained. But this hint of promise did not change much for their family. When I met Shlomo, they had just had their third child, a sweet brunette girl with her father's wide smile. Now, with three kids, Shlomo told me: "We have a mortgage, we have responsibility, we aren't playing around anymore. After all these years, we never really had time to build our own relationship. We don't have time to just be together. Now, after summer break and all the festivals. It has been very hard. Things have gone crazy. We are just too busy. We are not breathing."

Shlomo introduced me to his wife, Miriam, a few weeks later. Miriam told me how happy she was to become a mother but that she began to rethink her fertility trajectory after they had two children. She said:

I saw women who were already having their fourth child. They are amazing, they are my friends, but what it does to their bodies, ... to their children, to what they talk about.... I would look at the rabbi's wife who had nine children, and look at what she looked like and what her life looked like. I told Shlomo it scared me. You know, two more years like this and I am not sure if we will be able to navigate our life in any other direction. We didn't want to end up like that, so we moved.

I met Miriam and Shlomo at their new home in Jerusalem. As I knocked on the door, I could hear Miriam and Shlomo tidying up their house. They opened the door a few moments later and invited me to join them as they prepared a fresh pot of herbal tea. I brushed away a toy car as we sat down on their family-friendly sofa. I met them at the end of August, after two months when their kids were not attending childcare. They were so tired, I could hear it in their words and see it on their bodies. Miriam reflected on their choices:

When I look back at it, I realize how there are so many things we don't see. It is like a negative. You can see what there is, but you can't see what isn't there. This situation of parenting, birth . . . it doesn't enable me to see what the price is at that moment. What I am losing? What is not happening? I was in a very positive place. And now, I am looking at the negative. At what I don't have. I look at the damages. What it means to have three young children one after another. Everything that isn't happening will continue not happening. And I am not willing. I have chosen. Because all the things that aren't happening are starting to hurt me. I feel helpless. You can't get everything done. I keep on asking myself: Who is first? My husband? My children? The house? Work? My body? Who is first?

*\*\**

As I collected stories from Orthodox couples like Miriam and Shlomo, I noticed the growing ambivalence in their high-fertility dreams and long-standing commitment to make a large Jewish family. On top of struggles to constantly make ends meet, they were failing to create the romantic relationships they dreamed of and falling short of being the parents they believed their children deserved. Shlomo and Miriam were but one of many couples who shared their constant feelings of frustration as economic concerns, bodily strains, and professional advancement challenged the family dreams they shared at the beginning of their journey. Even though couples like Miriam and Shlomo described these as personal struggles,[2] these issues are deeply shaped by economic and structural changes in Israel's mode of "reproductive governance," aimed at limiting the high fertility rates among the religious population.[3]

Reproduction in Israel has always been political. Even before the State of Israel was formally established, Jews in Mandatory Palestine were fixated on what is often described as "womb wars," a sphere in which individual and collective survival were conflated. Since the establishment of the state in 1948, Israel has maintained a strong infrastructure that encourages procreation. This desire to increase the population is rooted both in the trauma of the Holocaust, which decimated nearly one-third of the world's Jewish population, such that the total number of Jews worldwide today has still not returned to what it was before World War II, and in concerns about maintaining the Jewish "nature" of the state. To secure a Jewish majority in Israel-Palestine, state interventions in private life were focused on the production of Jewish babies to win a demographic battle.

Today, however, there is a newly perceived "demographic threat" that must be governed by the Jewish state. Since the late 1990s, growing national concerns have shifted from a fixation on Jewish-Arab head counting to nationhood struggles over the future "face" of the Jewish state. Currently, Haredi (ultra-Orthodox) Jews in Israel have, on average, double the number of children had by Israel's nonreligious Jewish population, and they are making up an increasing proportion of the Israeli population. Demographic forecasts show that by 2065, Haredi Jews will constitute a third of Israeli's population (and will increase from 12 percent in 2020 to 32 percent in 2065), and for many, the most urgent demographic threat has become the growth of this Haredi sector.[4]

Israel today is thus navigating internal struggles over what kind of Jewish state it wants to be—a debate that is playing out through tensions over reproduction. Attempts to produce a particular kind of Jewish state have included discourses of reproduction, from allegations of forced contraception for Ethiopian immigrant women to denying surrogacy rights to gay men, capturing how fundamental reproductive logics are for promoting heterosexual and Ashkenazi Jewish births.[5] Yet, desires to reproduce the "Jewish state" extend beyond issues of race, ethnicity, or sexual orientation.

The Haredi sector today accounts for roughly 12 percent of Israel's population. Haredi Jews are a tightly knit group, often referred to as an enclave, and they maintain strict social and cultural boundaries.[6] The community's religious mores strive to adhere to the Hebrew Bible as well as a voluminous body of rabbinic literature, commentary, and rulings.[7] Haredi ultra-Orthodoxy is distinguished from other Jewish streams (Reform, Conservative, and Religious Zionist, among others). Compared with other Jewish denominations that offer different combinations of adherence to halacha (Jewish law) and embrace of "modern" lifestyles, including secular education, Haredim have a low level of workforce participation, as many of the men study full-time instead in religious institutions of higher learning (yeshivot).

In addition to concerns about the type of Jewish state Israel wants to be, there are thus economic concerns as well, with fears among some that "the Haredi Problem," as it is often referred to in public rhetoric, is creating circumstances that will "destroy Israel's economy." As Meirav Arlosoroff, a well-known economic reporter for *Haaretz* (a national newspaper known for its left-wing stance), put it recently: "We are walking towards bankruptcy."[8]

Moreover, most Haredi Jews are not Zionists,[9] and anxieties about the future "face" of the state are deeply linked to that Zionist ambivalence, which is mirrored in the exemption of Haredim from compulsory military service and abstention from national celebrations, such as Independence Day. These concerns signal how growing numbers of Haredi Jews pose threats not only to Israel's economy but also to the performance of Israeli citizenship and religion-state relations, which have been reflected in continuous ideological tugs-of-war in the Israeli Parliament and international relations. In a way, "the Haredi Problem" thus resonates with age-old issues, often framed as "the Jewish Question" in relation to the politics of Jewish belonging and citizenship.

In response, Israeli policy makers have attempted to manage the rapid increase in the ultra-Orthodox Jewish population, including through steep cutbacks in child benefits. The cutbacks, which were introduced at the beginning of the twenty-first century, functioned as economic sanctions designed to manage and reduce the rapid growth among Israel's ultra-Orthodox. In 2003, then Minister of Finance Benjamin Netanyahu led a capitalist reform of Israel's economic system. These radical changes included privatizing major Israeli businesses, cutting corporate income taxes and welfare payments, and, most relevant to this book, drastically reducing child allowances.[10] Netanyahu's official position, as he put it, was to "stop people from thinking that making children is work."[11]

I began my ethnographic research of reproductive decision-making among Orthodox (Dati) and ultra-Orthodox (Haredi) Jews in 2011, at the height of these tensions. In a community where contraception is considered taboo, I wondered, how will these policy changes affect the intimate lives of Israel's Orthodox Jews? This book examines how these changing discourses and public policies are reshaping the reproductive desires of Orthodox and ultra-Orthodox Jews in Israel, charting changes developing in the ideal of the large family among the Orthodox and exploring how these challenges to religious convictions are causing a sometimes painful process of "reorienting" desires to reproduce and have as many children as possible. The ethnography draws on stories from Orthodox and ultra-Orthodox couples that illuminate how hard their high-fertility dreams have become to achieve. It is an enormous financial challenge, not to mention a parenting and relationship one, to support the sorts of large families common in the community. With less government support for having children, competing secular models of "good" parenting, pressures on women's bodies and on couples' relationships, and an incipient feminist movement in Orthodox communities, I found "cracks" in couples' commitments—and their ability—to live up to moral, communal, and religious commitments to have as many children as possible.

I call these ambivalences "cracks" to highlight the painful gaps I found in the narratives and practices of my interlocuters between large-family ideals and their own lived realities. These cracks are painful because they embody the moments when ideals cannot be stretched any further and the many threads that hold life together are ripped apart. I often imagine that these cracks are what it feels like when a carpet you are standing on is forcefully drawn out from under your feet. Perceived in this way, a shrinking state infrastructure is a form of state violence. In keeping with contemporary anthropological writing, I conceptualize the state as an "assemblage of agents, mechanisms, institutions, ideologies and discourses" that are far from stable, coherent, or monolithic.[12] Building on this literature, I aim to tell a story about the shifting and conflicting desires of the state while focusing on the ways these desires bring forward new policies. In turn, I wish to understand the ways these shifting policies create cracks in the most intimate desires of the people I met.

While Orthodox Jews, and especially ultra-Orthodox men and women, are constantly represented in public discourse as being committed to developing large families, this book explores how Orthodox men and women have come to doubt whether (and how) to continue one of the pivotal religious commandments and communal ideals—populating the "promised land." On the one hand, having a large family is an important religious obligation and an internalized communal norm that has become a desire for Orthodox men and women. Yet, on the other hand, shifting forms of Israel's reproductive governance make the process of actualizing these high-fertility ideals and pressures almost unattainable.[13]

This book goes beyond the tendency to attribute religious reproduction to biblical commands to "be fruitful and multiply" by investigating how everyday religious people negotiate their reproductive desires in the midst of demographic shifts and anxieties in a pronatal Jewish state. Scholars have focused on the ways religious communities struggle with religious doubt, which often leads to defection.[14] In this book, I focus on how religious members critique, challenge, and reshape communal norms while remaining part of their communities. The Orthodox devotees portrayed here do not give up on their faith when confronted with religious doubt but instead reconfigure—or reorient—their desires. I draw on recent anthropological calls to study moments of doubt, while exploring not just pro-ceptive but also contraceptive desires around family formation, such as when to have children, how many, and at what cost.

In this book, I argue that cracks create conditions for new "ethical choreographies" and new voices to be heard.[15] I draw on queer theories of "orientation" to demonstrate how Orthodox desires are reshaped at the intersections of reproduction, religion, state, and politics. Analyzing the entanglement of personal and national desires offers a glimpse into Orthodox desires and how they are reoriented amid changing political and economic forces. Showcasing how Orthodox groups from a variety of backgrounds offer competing visions of secular Zionism, this ethnography offers fresh ways to see how notions of desire and promise are contested and changed. By highlighting cracks in patriarchal family ideals, we can see the powerful pronatalist logic that underlies Israeli religious reproduction in the so-called Jewish state.

The words used as the title of this book, the "state of desire," thus encompass multiple meanings. On the most basic level, they refer to a particular state—the State of Israel—that has continuously put concerted efforts into shaping the most intimate desires of its citizens. But, the state of desire is also a conceptual tool we can use to focus our attention on the sociopolitical conditionings of desire anywhere. According to this framework, states of desire are conditioned by a confluence of social, cultural, technological, political, and religious forces that shape individual and collective desire. Focusing on desire, instead of, say, ideology, action, or praxis, allows us to capture its temporality, which is shaped by specific political circumstances at a particular moment in time.

Highlighting the dynamic aspects of desire, this conceptualization refers to the ways states change their visions, which have a direct impact on the lives of citizens. As the State of Israel changes its desire(s), its citizens are compelled to reconfigure their most intimate family dreams. These transformations bring forward everyday uncertainties that religious people experience amid shifting state infrastructures. In the face of converging desires, creative ethical choreographies emerge and new ethics of decision-making are fashioned. Highlighting how these two states of desire—the individual's and the state's—are constantly intertwined, I show how reorienting desire is simultaneously a personal and communal project.

* * *

This book might make you feel uncomfortable. It employs queer theory to conceptualize the desires of heterosexual couples in one of today's most conservative religious contexts. My interlocutors, especially those who live in the West Bank, might also make you feel uncomfortable. In addition, whereas most anthropologists, especially Jewish ones, tend to be secular, I am an observant Jew. I am not ultra-Orthodox (and never was), my positionality is different from that of most other authors of ethnographies on the subject. This positionality shaped my encounters in the field, as well as the questions I ask and the theories I advance in this book. I am also a mother, which, as I discuss, was essential to my fieldwork, even more than my being an observant Jewish woman.

When I started working on this book, I was a student at the Hebrew University of Jerusalem, conducting ethnographic fieldwork among Haredi teenagers in a Bais Yaakov girls' seminary in Jerusalem.[16] I still remember the first time I heard a young Haredi teenager critique the obvious link between marriage and children. It was a chilly Tuesday morning when Racheli, one of the seminary students, got engaged. Class was canceled, and the entire student group celebrated together. After much singing and dancing, I took a step out of the classroom to catch a breath of air and overheard two teenagers chatting on a bench outside. "I can't believe Racheli is going to be the first one to become a mother!" one of the girls was squealing. The other girl laughed and said: "Who knows, she might decide to wait!"

I was taken by surprise by what I heard. Not only were these two girls speaking indirectly about contraception, a topic that is considered taboo in their communities, but I was surprised to hear that delaying a pregnancy was even thinkable—or enunciable—at their life stage. Large families are often considered one of the enduring commitments of Haredi Judaism, especially in Israel. Most couples are expected to have a child within one year of their marriage and would typically consider any other outcome a failure. While sitting on a rickety bench that chilly morning, I learned that this ethos may be changing.

Since overhearing these two teenagers challenging one of the most basic norms in their communities (while their friends were singing Jewish wedding songs inside), I have heard stories from many Orthodox couples about not being sure whether they wanted to have the large families like the ones they grew up in. This was big news.

* * *

When I began this project in 2011, my colleagues repeatedly laughed at me. "Contraception among Haredi Jews," they would say. "You will write the shortest book ever!" This remark reflected a common notion, that I too once shared, that ultra-Orthodox Jews always have many children and that this was not something that could change. My colleagues' teasing also reflected a dominant discourse and social judgment that while "normal" people planned their families properly, Haredi Jews have irresponsibly large families. This judgment was directly linked to assumptions about reproduction among Haredim, who are said to be blindly committed to procreation. Whereas "normal" people typically calculate the best time to have a child, Haredim just followed religious commandments without any hesitation.

It is for this reason that scholars have highlighted how pronatalist policies and social infrastructures shape every aspect of reproduction in Israel, but Haredi fertility is often treated as an exception. Perceived as an enduring religious commitment that is set in stone, Orthodox reproduction has been conceptualized as part of a siloed religious domain, one that has little or nothing to do with politics. Yet as the preceding discussion of demographic anxieties suggests, this too is changing.

In this book, I conceptualize reproduction as a biological and social process in which individual desires, technologies, and state policy are intertwined. My understanding of reproduction builds on the intellectual advancements of scholars of reproduction, especially Sarah Franklin, Faye Ginsburg, Marcia Inhorn, Heather Paxson, Rayna Rapp, and Marilyn Strathern, who have demonstrated how reproduction constructs almost every aspect of human life: gender, body, kinship, health and medicine, state politics, and inequalities associated with race, sexuality, disability, and nationality.[17] Reproduction, as Sarah Franklin has shown, "is itself a means of producing other things, other relationships, other values, or other identities."[18]

This book is inspired by the works of feminist scholars in the region—especially Susan Kahn, Daphna Birenbaum-Carmeli, Tsipy Ivry, Elly Teman, Yael Hashiloni-Dolev, Rhoda Kanaaneh, and Michal Raucher—who have shown how the centrality of reproduction in Judaism and Jewish-Israel culture shapes state policy, public discourse, and the lives of everyday people.[19] I also build on reproductive justice frameworks and settler-colonial readings of reproduction in Israel.[20] I have especially utilized ideas from Rhoda Kanaaneh's work that highlights the racialized and political tolls such policies take on Palestinian and Israeli-Arab reproduction.[21] Focusing on a different group of Israel's "Others,"[22] I show how Orthodox reproduction in Israel is best articulated through a narrative of state violence that continues to center on reproduction.

To understand the reorientation of Orthodox desires vis-à-vis changing state policies, I draw heavily on the concept of "reproductive governance," introduced by anthropologists Elizabeth Roberts and Lynn Morgan, which refers to the mechanisms through which different legislation, economic inducements, and moral discourse "produce, monitor, and control reproductive behaviors and population practices."[23] Reproduction discourses are increasingly framed through moral regimes that are used to "govern intimate behaviors, ethical judgments and their public manifestations."[24] Building on Michel Foucault's "regimes of truth" and Didier Fassin's notion of the "politics of life,"[25] this framework focuses on the evaluation of actions and ideologies as they are related to maintaining human continuity. To give a few examples, moral regimes in the context of reproduction may take shape through diverse sexual behaviors and identities, family formations, gendered division of labor, religious and spiritual commitments, and idealized forms of social reproduction (e.g., education or social security). To be clear, population control policies always mirror and produce ideological guideposts for what families should look like (even though we only see these as "producing ideology" during moments of "radical" or shifting policy, such as the one-child policy in China).

Reproductive governance is also shaped by the Foucauldian distinction between governance through sovereign—or state—power and biopower, which, by contrast, is how subjects come to govern themselves through intimate forms of self-surveillance and management. In this vein, this analytic lens examines subject-making within the context of moral regimes directed toward reproductive behaviors but also as fully entangled within political economy processes. As historians and feminist social theorists have noted, even though reproduction has been made to appear as an intimate and personal choice, it is fully entangled in the production of nation-states and economies. As Laura Briggs has argued: "There is no outside to reproductive politics, even though that fact is sometimes obscured."[26] It is in this sense that reproductive governance offers a useful guide for examining links between embodied moral regimes, national political strategies, and economic logics in Israel. Analyzing processes of intimate desire amid shifting reproductive governance, I draw on this concept to direct our attention to the ways reproduction is mobilized and activated at a particular moment in the history of the State of Israel.

In this book, I argue that after years of focusing on Jewish-Arab womb wars, the Israeli state has shifted its reproductive violence to inner-Jewish wars about the future face of the state. In *The Economization of Life*, Michelle Murphy offers a division between two forms of biopolitics—"quality" and "quantity." According to this distinction, the wave of eugenics that circulated in the early twentieth century was focused on quality, or, as she put it, "projects to govern life and death toward breeding better racial futures: more fit, more pure, more evolved, more uplifted races."[27] But, these quality-oriented politics switched to quantity biopolitics as neo-capitalist logics transformed "population" into a "problem that needed to be both represented and intervened in at the intersection of economics and biology."[28] Echoing Murphy's distinction, I show that in its current demographic "crisis," new desires of the state bring forward fresh strategies of quality biopolitics. By focusing on inner-Jewish womb wars, I do not intend to erase the violent history of reproductive politics in the region. On the contrary, I wish to open another front for analyzing state violence that continues to be driven by reproductive logics. In addition to the violence that is directed toward Palestinians, there are also other forms of power that are reproduced through Israel's reproductive policies, and examining them is an urgent task.[29]

This story is not unique to Israel or to Middle East conflicts. Religion plays a prominent role in reproductive politics around the globe, even if that fact is, at times, obscured. Consider the current Hindu-Muslim tensions in India, Evangelical abortion politics particularly in the United States, the fear of "Jihad wombs" in Germany, or President Erdogan's new pronatalist regime in Turkey.[30] Religion and reproductive politics are deeply intertwined through questions of righteousness and nationalist dreams of the future.

While scholars of reproductive politics have heavily analyzed race, gender, and nationalism,[31] they rarely attend to religion.[32] This book fills this lacuna and complements the surge of recent scholarship on reproductive politics, while highlighting the role religion plays within these assemblages of power. Ethnographers of the Middle East have robustly examined the intersection of religion and reproduction, but they have focused exclusively on the context of assisted reproduction, which reifies an image of religious men and women pursuing what Marcia Inhorn calls "quests for conception."[33] This book is thus a rare look at issues of contraception in the context of reproductive politics, beyond work on abortion, in vitro fertilization (IVF), surrogacy, and other reproductive technologies.[34] Focusing on contraception also offers fresh insights into the field of medical anthropology, which has overtly focused on advanced technologies while leaving "low-tech" areas of medicine understudied.[35]

My methodological approach explicitly focused on interviews with Orthodox and ultra-Orthodox couples to showcase the dilemmas that emerge between them, highlighting what I describe as the gendered shape of desire. Giving voice to men's desires and dilemmas around Orthodox family-making adds a fresh set of perspectives to the social study of reproduction, in which women's experiences are disproportionately centered. Further, examining the role of male desires and dilemmas around Orthodox family-making challenges hegemonic representations of Jewish-Israeli masculinity.

## Conceiving Israel's Pronatalist Infrastructure

On April 5, 2013, Roni, a thirty-two-year-old modern-Orthodox Jew, posted a picture on Facebook of a letter he found in the drawer of his late grandmother. Dating back to 1950, this letter celebrated the birth of her tenth child and included a gift of 100 lirot from the Israeli government, as was customary in the early years of the state. Roni's Facebook post was shared more than four hundred times, and, while many commentators had previously never heard of this state celebration of fertility, it provoked diverse responses.

Watching this thread unfold online, I noticed that some Israelis took pride in the state's recognition of women's reproductive labor; others were bothered by government celebration of women in state-building through fertility. Some commentators offered more details about Israel's "special" interest in making so many (Jewish) babies. Some compared this policy to other countries and their social and government interventions in the lives of individuals. I noticed the pain of parents who only wished the government would support them now, just as it had done in the past. One religious mother responded bitterly, "If only we would have such state-support now! All they do now is make it harder for us!"

What is the story of Israel's changing reproductive governance? And what can these shifts tell us about diverging desires shaped by religion, reproduction, and the state?

Departing from contemporary demographic anxieties of lowering total fertility levels in the United States and Europe,[36] Israeli women have produced higher total fertility rates than women in most industrialized countries in the Organisation for Economic Co-operation and Development (OECD). This divergence from global demographic anxieties (where total fertility rates are dropping) is directly linked to Israel's pronatalist ambitions—rooted, as we have seen, in post-Holocaust, Zionist, and religious ideologies.[37]

Looking at Jewish pronatalism from a historical perspective reveals that this stance was not always the case. Indeed, procreation holds supreme discursive importance in Judaism. Every one of the matriarchs in Genesis struggled with barrenness, cementing the "quest for conception" as one of the pillars of biblical narrative.[38] Yet, the religious obligation "to be fruitful and multiply" has continuously been reinterpreted by religious authorities and families alike.[39] According to feminist Jewish law scholar Ronit Irshai, most opinions in Jewish law on reproduction require a minimum of two children, ideally one of each sex.[40] Crucially, the obligation for reproduction falls on men, and hence from a position

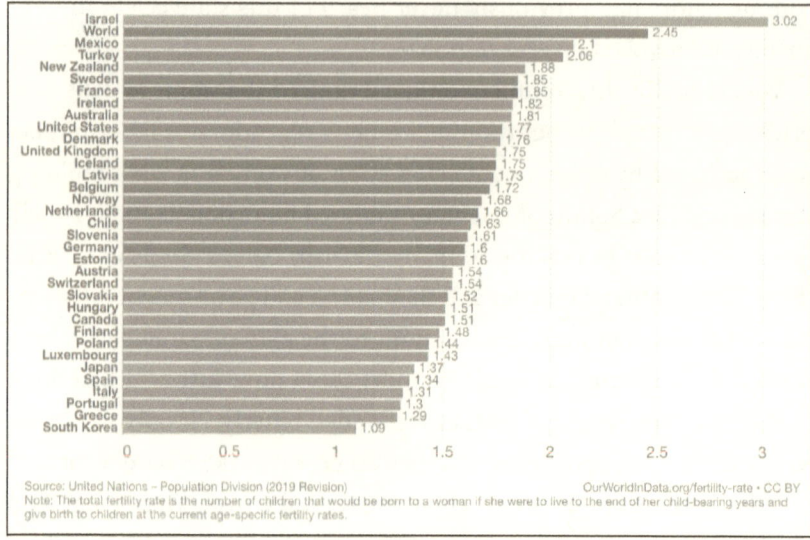

FIGURE 1.1. Fertility rate: Children per woman, 2019.

of Jewish law, women are exempt from the obligation to procreate.[41] Rabbinic positions around contraception are informed by a multilayered legal system of concerns that may be taken into consideration, such as physical and mental health, financial issues, and child welfare. There is, however, social and religious pressure to have large Jewish families that has been cultivated by a communal quest for Jewish survival during centuries of diaspora existence. When a couple is permitted to use birth control, they may only use methods that do not "waste seed."[42] Today, the Pill is the most preferred method whereas mechanical methods, like the condom, if allowed at all, are least preferred.

Yet, Jews did not always have large families. Historian Lilach Rosenberg-Friedman, who studied birth rate politics during the British Mandate in Israel-Palestine (1920–48), revealed that the birth rate of the Jewish community during the governance of the British Mandate declined steadily. At the eve of World War I, a typical Jewish family living in Ottoman Palestine had, on average, five children (with, as we will see, vast birth rate differences between Ashkenazi and Mizrahi Jews).

However, over the course of the British Mandate, from 1920 to 1948, the birth rate declined steadily. By 1941, the Hebrew press reported that "among the Jews, a fourth child is an exception. Even a third and second child are rare."[43] This resonates with findings collected in 1944 by Roberto Bachi, an Israeli statistician and demographer (who founded the Israeli Central Bureau of Statistics), showing that half of all Jewish families were childless or had only one child, a quarter had two children, and only a quarter had more than two children.[44] Although Bachi attempted to warn the Jewish population of this "collective suicide," as he put it, birth rates continued to plummet.

Given the anticipated growth of the Arab population, the pre-state leadership of the Jewish residents in Palestine (the Yishuv) concluded that it was imperative for each family to have at least three children to guarantee the Yishuv's Jewish future and a majority in the future state. The Yishuv leaders looked at the different policies Western countries began to adopt to encourage higher birth rates. At that moment in time, demographic panic was evident in many European countries, a preexisting anxiety that was exacerbated in the period between the two world wars.[45] Democracies and dictatorships alike were intervening in the lives of individuals, most notably in Germany, Britain, Russia, and France. The subordination of reproductive rights to national needs was especially evident in the nationalist and fascist regimes such as Nazi Germany, Mussolini's Italy, and Franco's Spain, but other countries also placed national birth rates at the center of public discourse. Three primary strategies were implemented by different countries: anti-abortion measures, education, and economic incentives.

Yet, the pre-state Yishuv was still only a voluntary public association with limited ability to enforce any decisions its leadership made. These leaders all agreed that high fertility rates were a national goal and were searching for the best ways to push for a local campaign to promote Jewish birth rates. In fact, as Lilach Rosenberg-Friedman put it, "The Yishuv's grappling with the birth rate issue and its attempts to shape a systematic policy with regard to it was mortar in the construction of the future state."[46] At first, these efforts were pushed forward by individuals, but at the beginning of 1943, after the Yishuv leadership confirmed that Nazis systematically murdered Jews, a new wave of encouragements were introduced. In addition to private initiatives, special committees were established to address the birth rate "problem." Many of these initiatives never saw the light of day, but one project, the prize for mothers of large families began in 1944, donated by an anonymous dentist, created public awareness and appreciation of motherhood. In its first format, this was a prize given in appreciation of mothers' effort to have children, regardless of the numbers of children a woman actually had. This prize was the earliest version of the official prize initiated by David Ben Gurion, the first prime minister of Israel, which, as mentioned earlier, offered an economic award to women who contributed to the state effort by having at least ten children.

Out of all the different pronatalist initiatives, the establishment of the national Committee on Birthrate Problems in 1943, was the most significant. This committee began "a systematic action plan against the distressing decline in the birthrate," as declared in its official statement.[47] The committee started to collect data on birth rates, abortions, and more. Because abortions were already prohibited by law (but practiced widely in private), the committee decided to focus its energy on increasing public awareness and devoting all resources to creating economic incentives for larger families. With few economic resources at hand, public education had to be the primary action, which would be followed by an economic program. In his book, written in 1944, Yitzhak Kanievsky, explains that "without knowing they could afford to feed, clothe, and educate their children properly, the prospect of a second or third child would seem to most Yishuv families a perilous rather than a joyous prospect."[48] Thus, the committee promoted laws aimed at transforming childbearing from being perilous to joyful, through public education as well as assistance through economic incentives. These suggestions included guaranteed maternity leave, breastfeeding breaks, tax and salary benefits for fathers, salary supplements for families with children, discounts for the cost of housing, and an aid package for new mothers.

After the establishment of the state in 1948, Israel continued to develop an elaborate pronatal infrastructure aimed at ensuring a Jewish majority over a growing Arab minority population. In practice, many of the pronatalist incentives suggested by the Committee on Birthrate Problems were implemented only years later, by the Israeli government, with paid maternity leave as the first social benefit installed by the state. This was the first in many state policies established to promote pronatalism: child allowances, remuneration in proportion to number of children (in the public sector, between 1940 and 1950), special tax reductions for employed mothers, and national awards for "heroine mothers" who delivered their tenth child and "to families blessed with many children," as the committee put it.[49]

Since these pronatalist infrastructures were put into place, Israel's model of reproductive governance continues to heavily fund childcare and family benefit systems, paternalist abortion policies, and subsidized access to assisted reproductive technologies that promote heterosexual reproduction.[50] While these policies were mainly geared toward the Jewish population, in effect, they applied to all Israeli citizens. In 1968, the government established the Demographic Center; its goal, as defined in its founding document, was stated as follows: "Carrying out a reproductive policy intended to create a psychologically favorable climate that will encourage and stimulate natality; an increase in natality in Israel being crucial for the future of the whole Jewish people."[51] Since then, the Israeli government continued to expand publicly funded pronatalist incentives: obstetric follow-up, maternity care, child allowances, and fertility treatments. In the labor market, economic incentives were also introduced, including mother-friendly taxation and laws to protect pregnant and working mothers. In parallel, researchers have pointed to the insufficiency of sex education and contraception in Israel.

Hence, even though Jewish natality and the centrality of the Jewish family can be traced to biblical times, pronatalist responses to the

Nazi devastation and threat of extermination, together with the Zionist ideology of demographic threats, all contributed to the enlargement of the Jewish nation as an important aspect of nation-building. Reproduction, as Daphna Birenbaum-Carmeli and Yoram Carmeli put it, "became a sphere of convergence between the private and the political, in which individual survival was virtually equated with the survival of the collectivity."[52]

## The Racial Politics of Jewish Reproduction

While Israeli Jewish pronatalism, at first sight, offers an image of unbound and monolithic high fertility, the picture is actually much more complicated (and stratified). Before exploring this history, a brief note about race, ethnicity, and religion in the Jewish context is necessary. As historian Leora Batnitzky has shown, in the eighteenth century Judaism was transformed from a multifaceted fusion of cultural, social, ethnic, and theological forces into a "religion" in the modern nation-state.[53] This Protestant-inspired shift was embraced by leading Jewish thinkers in the nineteenth and twentieth centuries as a possible solution for a particularist people who wished to affirm the authority of God and also lead civic lives in modern Europe.

Framing Judaism as *only* a religion positions Judaism as nonpolitical. However, the birth of Zionist ideology, amid nationalist and anti-Semitic discourses of Jewishness in Eastern Europe, created new political circumstances.[54] As Yaakov Yadgar has recently demonstrated, pre-state Zionism put forward notions of Jewishness that are primarily a matter of "blood" and "biology." According to Yadgar, "The defining, foundational element shaping the very core of this Jewish nationalism, then, is not a sense of a dialogue with some normative tradition and history (these will surely come into the picture in some readings of the Zionist idea, but only secondarily so), but an a priori sense of some so-called natural and biological determinant of Jewish identity."[55] Yadgar shows how the "biological" Jews (as opposed to Judaism) are now defined not by "what they do (or should do, aspire to do, etc.) but by what they are." While pre-Zionist notions commonly referred to Jews as part of a "family," forming this narrative as part of a political ideology in a context of a modern nation-state came with new connotations and politics.

This reconceptualization implied that the survival of Judaism, which has worried Jews for generations, was transformed to the survival of Jews. To put it simply, Israel became "only," or "simply," a vision of a state of Jews (not Judaism). This shift, in effect, introduced a new politics dedicated to the preservation of "biological," "racial," or "ethnic" Jews (terms that, as we will see, do not latch on simply to the Jewish-Israeli context). In addition, the diversity of Jewish traditions that immigrant communities brought with them was viewed by state elites as a threat to national unity. The violent state project of the "melting pot" viewed these diverse projects of Jewish life as objects that must be erased in order to create a new state.

It is worth noting here that historically, Jews have been divided among multiple ethnic groups, with the two most notable being the Ashkenazim and the Sephardim (often conflated as Mizrahim).[56] These two groups have some distinct religious practices and traditions that are associated with their ancestries, which is why, even today, Israel has two chief rabbis—one who is Ashkenazi and the other Sephardi. Ashkenazim (from the Hebrew word for Germany [Ashkenaz in singular, Ashkenazim in plural]), trace their roots to central and Eastern Europe while Sephardim trace their roots to a variety of places, spanning from Spain to the Middle East to Central Asia. The word "Mizrahi" means "east" in Hebrew but is often used interchangeably with "Sephardi" (meaning "Spanish" in Hebrew). Because many Sephardim who were expelled from Spain migrated east and settled in different locations in the Middle East and North Africa, Mizrahim and Sephardim tend to share similar religious customs and traditions. In the context of modern Israel's history, Sephardi/Mizrahi Jews have been discriminated against in various ways as part of the "melting pot" project. This erasure process took a particular ethnic form with its own reproductive logic, including engaged attempts to reduce Mizrahi fertility.

During the Yishuv period, small families were mainly an Ashkenazi phenomenon, in contrast to Mizrahi families, who had an average of four to five children. Yemenite families were singled out in public policy as having record large families. As one newspaper claimed: "They are the only community that strictly observed the commandment to be fruitful and multiply."[57] In addition, the Old Yishuv, which primarily meant Ashkenazi Haredim, who in general opposed the State of Israel and have continued to live in the four holy cities Jerusalem, Safed, Hebron, and Tiberias, were also known for their high birth rates. In 1945, five women were awarded a procreation prize (like Roni's grandmother mentioned earlier), three of whom were Mizrahi and two of whom were Ashkenazi women of the Old Yishuv. As we can see, birth rates clearly defined the differences between the Old Yishuv and the New Yishuv.

This distinction resonates with anthropologist Rhoda Kanaaneh's findings that birth control practices and smaller family sizes were a sign of modernity in Israel-Palestine.[58] This distinction was deeply intertwined with Jewish racial politics as well. Yali Hashash has shown how in the 1950s and 1960s an association was observed between Mizrahi Jews, economic deprivation, and high fertility. According to these studies, high fertility was associated with the "backwardness" and "Arabness" of Mizrahi Jews, which was meant to be rectified by (Ashkenazi) Zionism.[59] Smadar Lavie has shown that Ashkenazi Zionist family experts reinvented motherhood and glorified it, but "only those at the crux of the Zionist ethos were able to be part of this. Others thought eugenically incapable of participation included Palestinians, Sephardim, Jewish immigrants from the Balkans and Muslim countries, and the ultra-Orthodox Ashkenazim whose majority was anti-Zionist."[60]

These Jewish racial politics not only were part of stigmatized discourses regarding Mizrahi reproduction but also were grounded in official policy. According to the formal declaration of "the Demographic Campaign," its activities were meant to encourage "families with two children to increase their families to 3–4 children, and advise large families on family planning." This dual and racial population control reveals that while Israel's early reproductive discourse primarily aimed for encouraging Jewish natality, there were also anti-natalist undercurrents that equated large families with racial backwardness and deprivation.[61] As Joseph Meir, the former head of Israel's largest health fund, put it in 1952: "We have no interest in the tenth or even the seventh child of the poor Mizrahi families ... we must pray for the second child of the families of the intelligentsia."[62] Unsurprisingly, among Mizrahi Jews, total fertility rates were significantly reduced from 5.7 children on average in 1955 to just over 3 in the 1970s. This rapid change has also been echoed in hushed stories about Ashkenazim stealing Yemenite babies to bring them up in better circumstances.[63]

Orthodox Jews, though, flourished in Israel's pronatal infrastructure. In a sense, the growth of "religious" Jews is perceived, primarily by Israel's secular elite, as fostering too much "Jewishness" in the "state of the Jews." Although Orthodox Jews in Israel are racially and ethnically diverse, Haredim, in particular, are often racialized. Similar to the ways in which Su'ad Kahbeer describes how Islam in the United States is often coded as "Black," religion can become raced.[64] This does not mean it is equated with blackness or with other kinds of discriminations other ethnicities face in Israel, but the category of "Haredi" in Israel often functions like a racial category that is subject to stigma, government policing, and, as we will see, particular biopolitics, which have ushered in a new era of reproductive governance.

## Israel's New Reproductive Logic

Why has the rapid growth of the Haredi Jewish population been met with such heightened anxiety by Israeli policy makers? Most Israeli Jews define themselves as part of one of the following groups: secular, traditional, Religious Zionist, or Haredi. Both Haredim and religious Zionists self-define as Orthodox in terms of Jewish law observation, but they differ socially and ideologically. These differences are most clear in two key ways. First, while Haredi ideology usually rejects Zionism, Religious Zionism embraces the Zionist movement as the harbinger of religious redemption. Second, Religious Zionists attempt to combine adherence to halacha with a modern lifestyle that includes secular education and army service. However, as mentioned earlier, Haredim do not enlist in the Israeli army and have a low level of workforce participation, as many men devote their lives to Talmudic studies in religious seminaries.[65]

In practice, the Haredi sector consists of multiple groups, each with its own religious leaders (rabbis), teachings, and observances. This populace can be loosely divided into the Lithuanian yeshiva-based (Torah learning) communities, the Hasidic dynasties, and Mizrahi Haredim. Differences aside, all the sectors' members are easily identified by their more or less shared dress code: black hats and dark suits for men and similarly colored ankle-length skirts, long sleeves, and head coverings for women.

In contrast to other Haredi communities across the globe, the post-Holocaust Israeli branch was originally intended to be a quietist society charged with a historic mission to perpetuate the "age-old" Jewish tradition that was nearly wiped out by the Nazis.[66] To this end, the community's founders sequestered the flock and its "sacred" culture within enclaves with the objective of shielding them from what they considered to be the liberal, depraved, and spiritually corruptive influences of Western civilization. During the mid-twentieth century, various ultra-Orthodox streams publicly opposed the founding and existence of a Jewish state. Consistent with their ideology of passively waiting for God to usher in the messianic era, the vast majority of Haredim rejected (at least in public) Zionism, secularism, and all other proactive models, both before or after the establishment of the state. The most glaring exceptions were demonstrations against perceived violations of major religious tenets or the status quo between the country's secular and observant Jewish citizens, such as heated rallies against the opening of Jerusalem's first public swimming pool in the late 1950s. The Haredi ethos

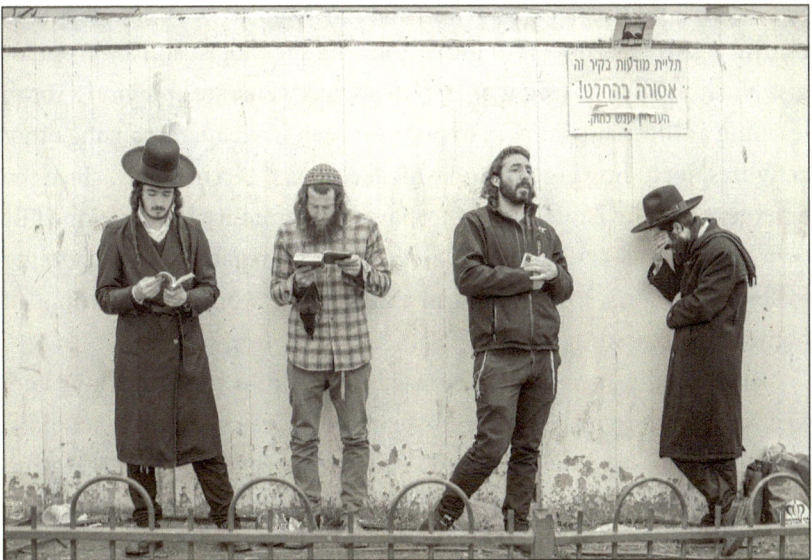

FIGURE I.2. Four praying men of different denominations. Photo by Avishag Shaar-Yashuv.

of Talmudic erudition and mitigating temporal concerns was sharply at odds with the fledgling Jewish state's secular and nationalist symbols, especially that of the productive and self-dependent Zionist worker or the self-sacrificing Hebrew warrior. In addition to their ideological rejection of Zionism, Haredim deemed Israeli aggressiveness to be coarse, and initially refrained from partaking in the affairs of the state, politics, the military, and the labor market.[67]

Upon Israel's establishment, the community's leaders introduced a new strain of ultra-Orthodox piety. Unlike the Jewish education system in prewar Eastern Europe in which only a few gifted young men had been chosen to pursue full-time Talmudic studies, all Haredi men were now slated for a path of erudite seclusion from the temporal world for the purpose of instituting what Menachem Friedman has coined a "society of learners."[68] From that point on, the Lithuanian community deemed the all-male yeshiva to be the only institution capable of defending and preserving the enclave.

Research on ultra-Orthodox male piety has demonstrated just how central yeshiva learning is to the sector.[69] As sociologist and anthropologist Nurit Stadler has shown, Haredi society venerates religious Torah learning as the main pathway to piety for men while marginalizing other activities, including employment-related ones.[70] Accordingly, since the emergence of the Israeli state, the Haredi community has developed its own educational system that is made up of segregated K–12 schooling for boys and girls, followed by an extensive network of institutions of higher religious study for men.[71]

Very broadly speaking, Haredi schools aim to prepare youngsters for their gender-specific roles in society—males as religious scholars, and females as breadwinners and domestic caregivers. For this reason, STEM (science, technology, engineering, and mathematics) subjects are sparsely taught in ultra-Orthodox schools, and most male students do not learn science beyond fifth or sixth grade (eleven or twelve years old). In the past, the state's efforts to introduce basic scientific learning into the curriculum were repelled by political pressure. However, over the past two decades, minimal core studies have been gradually introduced via a number of school reforms, alongside progressive changes in the educational sphere.[72] Scholars have also noted growing Haredi participation in the workforce, including the integration of some Haredi women into the high-tech industry.[73] These have been largely driven by the high poverty rates in Haredi society and by government cuts to welfare payments.

As Haredi fertility rates continue to grow, Haredi ambivalence toward Zionism, the limited levels of secular education in Haredi schools, and their vast majority exemption from compulsory military service created much of the demographic anxiety discussed earlier. The steep cutbacks in child benefits introduced at the beginning of the twenty-first century were met with anger by Haredi politicians (e.g., "We won't forgive wicked Netanyahu," promised ultra-Orthodox Knesset member Aryeh Deri), who struggled to restore child allowances for over a decade. This reproductive logic is also heavily driven by growing neoliberal and capitalist regimes. Today, after years of Israel pioneering assisted reproduction, existing biocapital is now being directed toward cutting-edge biogenetic research, positioning Israel as one of the leading countries in stem cell research.[74] As Israel's state policy shifts from pronatal incentives toward the creation of a neo-capitalist, high-income high-tech start-up nation, this policy change effects the lives and desires of its citizens.

## Reproductive Politics and Religion

In response to the expanding use of advanced technologies within reproductive medicine around the turn of the twenty-first century, anthropologists of reproduction considered what role religion played within encounters in high-tech biomedicine. Scholars have observed how religion frequently enters the lab or clinic in ways that render distinctions between the so-called sacred and profane difficult to discern.[75] Elizabeth Roberts, in her ethnography *God's Laboratory*, shares how clinicians would pray before transferring the IVF embryo into the woman's body ("God, allow me to select good embryos") or would "touch a crucifix that hung from the incubator in a sterile plastic bag and again make the sign of the cross."[76] These examples demonstrate how the scientific and divine intermingle among clinicians who deliver hope via technological interventions.[77]

Scholars have also examined how people of different faith traditions developed strategies for integrating technological innovations into their religious visions of the world.[78] These works have particularly highlighted how religious leaders offer creative interpretations of religious texts to incorporate advanced technologies into existing religious legal codes.[79] While this scholarship focuses on theological and legal strategies, anthropologist Marcia Inhorn puts particular emphasis on the lived realities and practices of religious men and women. For the past two decades, Inhorn has shown the convergences and divergences between "official" interpretations of Islam and "unofficial" discourses and practices of local peoples.[80] In Islam, third-party gamete donation is prohibited because donor technologies are considered immoral. Nevertheless, Inhorn has shown that regardless of these restrictive fatwas (Islamic rulings of law), third-party donations are indeed used by Muslim men and women. While men do not want to donate sperm because this would trouble kinship patterns, donor eggs are used secretly. In her work, Inhorn brings together Arthur Kleinman's concept of "local moral worlds" and Rayna Rapp's "moral pioneering" to go beyond the Euro-American emphasis and highlight "what is at stake for ordinary Muslims as they attempt to make reproductive decisions in a way that is morally satisfying and consistent with local religious norms."[81]

Inhorn's works spurred a wave of research examining how technologies were adopted and translated by different regions in the Middle East, especially in Iran, Lebanon, and Turkey.[82] While these ethnographers of the Middle East have helped us understand the complexities of constructing local moral worlds vis-à-vis changing technologies, they have typically focused on assisted reproduction. By maintaining this focus, though, reproduction is constantly constructed as a mission that is almost blindly pursued. By analyzing contraception, I build on these insights to consider different, albeit coexisting, desires around family formation. Without this type of analysis, we risk framing reproduction, especially in the Middle East, as a project merely consisting of "reproductive desires" while marginalizing the multiplicities of desires and failures that are part and parcel of reproductive decision-making. Shifting the focus of analytical inquiry, I ask: What are the particular ethical anxieties contraceptive technologies bring to the table?

Family planning is a site for negotiating significant social concepts such as femininity, masculinity, culture, modernity, nationalism, and race. As anthropologist Rhoda Kanaaneh put it: "Family planning is now part of the social processes in which these concepts are daily defined, changed, and redefined in people's lives; in which gender is configured, communities are imagined, and boundaries of the modern are drawn."[83] In contrast to much feminist inquiry focused on the developments and consequences of "high-tech" reproductive technologies, focusing on contraception as a site for nation-building has been helpful to illuminate everyday decisions as sites for political resistance. This is not, of course, unique to the Middle East. While conducting ethnographic research on family planning in Greece, Heather Paxson has shown how ethics are formed through reproductive decision-making, especially during times of change. She writes, "As ethics is inextricable from historical context, it cannot be untethered from political control or, for that matter, political struggle."[84]

Feminist scholars have gone the farthest at highlighting how birth control has been constantly linked to projects of political governance and inequality as a technology of state biopolitics. Kanaaneh has shown how, in the Israel-Palestine context, Palestinian clinics doled out contraception, while it was much harder to get access to contraception in Jewish clinics. Her work ushered in new ways to think about reproduction in Israel-Palestine while utilizing settler-colonial frameworks. This intervention has highlighted the importance of unpacking Zionist logics and politics while examining reproduction as a central site for state violence.

While scholars have vividly shown how these parallel systems of racialized population control affect the everyday lives and decisions of Palestinians and Arab-Israelis, we still do not know very much about the other side of this state policy, especially in terms of contraception. Based on my findings, I argue that these are two sides of the same (stratified) reproductive logic. Family planning, as noted earlier, does not receive state support in Israel. Unlike fertility treatments, which are heavily funded by the state, contraception is not part of basic medical services, which in other areas of medicine are heavily supported by the Israeli government. Susan Kahn has noted that Israeli health officials explain that this "lacuna" is due to lack of funding, which, as we know, is solely directed toward making babies. Relatedly, abortions, while legal, are subsidized only for those under the age of seventeen or over forty, or, in other words, those whose pregnancies present a health liability for either mother or the child or were the result of rape or incest.[85] The reproductive logic organizing these state policies is clear in both contraception and abortion regulations—the state makes it extremely difficult to go against the pronatalist infrastructure.

In examining Orthodox Jews' ethical choreographies of family planning in Israel, I aim to open up another front for examining reproductive (in)justice. Not only has family planning been left unexamined, but Orthodox contraception is an even more uncommon topic of consideration. This academic lacuna, especially in the Middle East context, is primarily linked to a tradition within anthropology of religion that often studies religion through questions of dogma instead of doubt. In the context of reproduction, scholars have tended to ignore the complexities of birth control because of their (assumed) enduring commitments to religious obligations.

## Dogma versus Doubt

From its establishment as a field of study, anthropology of religion has been deeply embedded in the process of constructing terms like "religion," "religiosity," and "spirituality" as distinct and separate realms of human life.[86] This secular process of separation and demarcation has created many analytical problems, one of which I wish to address here. Framing religion and members of religious communities as separate entities, anthropologists focus their analysis as an attempt to make sense of these "religious entities." Influential works by Talal Asad and Saba Mahmood, for example, may be perceived as complex projects analyzing religious members' technologies of self while trying to make these processes legible to outsiders.[87] In other words, anthropologists were socialized to tell a story about how things (surprisingly) work.

While this seems to be a constructive route to take, I argue that it has created a problematic trajectory. On the one hand, Mahmood's project of making religious women's choices digestible to feminist or liberal critique has been highly influential, inspiring scholars to rethink religious agency. On the other hand, rereading Mahmood's account of religious women more critically reveals a limited picture of other aspects of these women's lives. Critiquing such studies for constructing a normative and harmonious picture of religious life, scholars have argued that "struggle, ambivalence, incoherence and failure, must also receive attention in the study of everyday religiosity."[88] In other words, they are begging us to stop telling a story of how things (always) work.

Amid this turn to study struggles and doubt in religious contexts, Ayala Fader's *Hidden Heretics* is particularly helpful.[89] Drawing on her fieldwork among Hasidic double-lifers in New-York, Jews who continue to live a religious life while doubting their faith in secret, Fader's ethnographic attention to life-changing doubt complicates conceptions of how anthropologists should study religious lives and subjectivities. Whereas most research on religious doubt focuses on those who have left the fold, Fader offers a compelling account of the ethical and emotional dilemmas that arise by living a secret heretical life while publicly continuing a performance of stringent religious life.

While Fader's account of the particular experiences of double-lifers is instrumental in developing a more nuanced account of different types of doubt, we still need to understand how struggles appear in the lives of religious men and women who are not considering leaving the fold. Sociologist Katie Gaddini, for example, shows how Evangelical women stay in male-dominated churches even though they are marginalized in these contexts.[90] Gaddini's study examines how hard it is for single women to stay in Evangelical communities, while highlighting the emotional tolls these women pay. In a similar vein, the point that I make in this book is that religious subjectivity is not in or out—believer or nonbeliever. Instead of this Protestant framing of religion as belief, I argue that there are all kinds of ways that religious subjects navigate lived experience versus some kind of ideal, whether from religious texts or parenting magazines.

Times of uncertainty are a fertile ground to "unravel the ways in which convictions gain and lose their force" at historical moments or across the individual's life course.⁹¹ Even though scholars have focused on the ways religious communities struggle with religious doubt and defection,⁹² I focus here on how religious members critique and reshape communal norms while remaining part of their communities. Emphasizing the stratified ways individual members critique communal norms, I provide a vivid and complicated account of how Jewish men and women struggle with, question, and debate the meaning of reproduction in contemporary Israel.

Studying the effects of shifting policies on Orthodox Jews (who believe they are continuing traditions that are far from the reach of the state) builds on an intellectual legacy of studying socioreligious minority groups as part of fluid relationships with the particular societies in which they live.⁹³ But how far will this tolerance go? Ben Kasstan has shown how ultra-Orthodox Jews in the United Kingdom are treated as a "hard to reach" group that must be managed "differently" by the state.⁹⁴ Yet, the governance of Jewish populations and bodies in the United States and the United Kingdom is vastly different as these groups continue to live at the margins of the state. As changing demographic futures threaten to shift the minority-majority balance among Jews in Israel, reproductive desires transform and new modes of reproductive governance are introduced to the public sphere. Hence, the structurally precarious position that religious minorities occupy in contemporary Israel and the particular shape this inequality takes are historically specific.⁹⁵ Even though my research provides insights from ethnographies of Orthodox life around the globe, the governance of Jewish populations and bodies in the Israeli context offers particular challenges. As the state engages with anxieties about its population growth, biopolitics are utilized to manage Israel's religious minority populations.⁹⁶

To analyze the cracks created by these shifting demographic anxieties, I draw on Sara Ahmed's work on desire, even though initially this theoretical use might seem unintuitive or inappropriate.⁹⁷ While desire has constantly been a main focus in psychological theory, Ahmed approaches the cultural aspects of shaping desire and its discontents. Her work offers a unique theory to capture how the queer body is perceived as a "failed orientation," while highlighting a process of reorientation that emerges from this moment of failure.[98] In what follows, I draw on this queer theory of orientation to characterize how men and women fail to live up to communal norms of large families as well as the ethical choreographies of reorientation these failures entail. I am well aware of the uneasiness that comes from my theoretical choice, and here I offer a brief reflection on my theory politics.

Anthropology, as Matei Candea argues, "has built itself around comparison."[99] While anthropologists have produced various versions (and visions) of the comparative method, on the most basic level it entails a positioning of case study x and case study y in parallel in order to draw out differences and similarities. This is how we can study ballerinas in Nepal by comparing them to a theory developed by Marcel Mauss in France or based on Mary Douglas's observations of the Lele in Kasai.[100]

Nevertheless, in the development of the field of anthropology, different theories were used to understand different "types" of people. Even as anthropological theory attempts to shift away from colonial modes of theorizing, we are still left with a legacy that entails various degrees of theoretical "othering." These constantly reveal how the ability to take a case study and generalize is historically and culturally situated. In addition, different subfields have produced particular traditions for studying specific phenomena. In the context of religion, this "theory bubble" means not only that anthropologists are expected to refer to particular theorists (say Talal Asad or Saba Mahmood, as I did earlier), but that this bubble simultaneously delineates what *should not* be typically used to study religious subjectivities and experiences.

As a result, when I explain that I use queer theory to conceptualize Orthodox desire, eyebrows are often raised. This surprise typically stems from two different directions of objection. The first objection is linked to a hegemonic intellectual trajectory in which there are conventional theories that have been developed to study particular aspects of religious subjectivity, and the assumption is that we should stick to them. In other words, the experience of religious life is so particular that we should continue to use (and produce) theories that are particular to religious experiences. The second reason for resistance is also linked to ideas about particularity but refers to the singularity of cisgender desire. At the core of this critique is a notion that queer desire is unique, rooted in a particular history of violence and cultivated as a response to it. Hence, because of this particularity it would not "make sense" to apply queer theory to the understanding of heterosexual desire.

In all these objections, we can detect an "epistemological purity" that confounds the contours of comparison. This purity is not only epistemological but also based on political assumptions that have a stake in keeping separate the theories about how subjectivity is made and experienced. While I understand where these objections are coming from, I argue that sometimes we need to go beyond these intellectual confinements. In my case, I acknowledge these theory politics and still think that we can learn much from comparing two contexts that seem, at first glance, as if they are worlds apart.

I noted in trying to conceptualize the cracks that emerged between the desire to have a large family and the everyday challenges of actualizing these dreams that these experiences resonated deeply with Ahmed's theory of queer orientation. Ahmed's theory eloquently captures "how the queer body becomes a failed orientation," as they follow nonbinary lines of desire. On the most basic level, both queer people and the Haredi men and women I studied felt they were not able to continue along the path everyone else is on (and is expected to be on).

The context of reproduction also highlights a more specific similarity. Much of queer "failure" is linked to futuristic ideals about biological reproduction and the production of a heterosexual family. Comparing queer failure to "achieve" this perceived "natural" life course, in the Orthodox context, highlights how biological reproduction is conceived as "natural," often substantiated in ethical discourses of righteousness. Thus, comparing the struggles faced by individuals in both of these groups highlights how hard resistance to so-called natural reproductive trajectories actually is. While the "failure" of queer desire pushes us to rethink the sociocultural invention of the heterosexual family as a natural desire, it also pushes us to think about the large Jewish family as a social product of a particular time and place, situated in particular pronatal discourses, practices, and theologies. In other words, by studying the two cases in parallel, we can draw out the social construct of both desires, as well as the painful process entailed in resistance.

Putting these case studies into conversation also reveals very explicit differences. First, while Orthodox defiance of social reproductive norms is met with massive social pressure and local modes of governance, queer desire has been subjected to a history of violent legal persecution. In my comparison of these cases, I do not mean to play down the severity of this violence. But I do draw on this history to learn how different types of desire are governed, and how these can change in different times and places. My ethnographic insights also advance Ahmed's phenomenology by showcasing a particular process of reorientation that emerges as people resist age-old social structures while aspiring to make good lives.

This unorthodox analysis is important for transporting Jewish studies and the anthropological study of religion, which has predominantly taken for granted the desires of religious people. This book shows that Orthodox desire is not reoriented only when the Orthodox decide to leave the fold. Further, anthropologists of religion who study doubt or uncertainty generally work at the individual level. By highlighting national, social, and economic infrastructures, I show how desire is shaped amid particular moments in history. In this vein, this case study allows us to look at a moment of ethical alignment of a society immersed in doubt. By focusing on family-making, this book also offers a unique perspective on religious doubt that is simultaneously personal and national.

## Studying Orthodox Desire: Methods and Tools

The initial stages of this research project were paved with many methodological challenges that needed to be addressed carefully. First, an attitude of silence with respect to sexuality exists among Israeli Orthodox Jews.[101] This realm of life is governed by strict rules and intrusive monitoring: boys and girls are partitioned from a young age, and sartorial modesty is tightly enforced (that said, discrepancies in the level of gender separation can be viewed as hallmarks of each group). I wondered: How can I find couples who would be willing to discuss such intimate topics with me? Even if I am able to find participants, how does one create a comfortable and inviting setting to enable couples to share topics that are almost unspeakable? How do I find the right words to open up a conversation? Merely using the ("secular" and rational) words "family planning" would certainly serve as a conversation stopper. Furthermore, because this conversation would include critique of customary norms, it would most likely entail emotions like guilt and failure. How does one create an interview setting that is not an ideological picture but that enables couples to share their doubts, struggles, and failures?

I also knew that collecting both women's and men's stories was crucial to this study. Yet, as a self-identifying female researcher, I wondered how I could find Orthodox men who would feel comfortable to share their thoughts with me. In a gender-segregated world, how was I going to find men who would be able to speak to me about such intimate topics?

To overcome these challenges, I utilized a creative and flexible research method and gained access to personal accounts of Orthodox desire. This book draws on five years of extensive, creative, and flexible multisited ethnographic research conducted in Israel, followed by continuous surveying of this field. Between 2011 and 2016, I surveyed over fifty communal gatherings, conferences, and classes on reproduction and the Jewish family, held by organizations affiliated with Haredi (ultra-Orthodox), Dati (Religious Zionist), and Hardal (national-Haredi) groups. As I attended conferences and classes regarding reproduction, I was surprised to find members from across the entire spectrum of Israeli Orthodoxy. I learned that these sites were nonsectorial spaces through which Orthodox Jews (especially women) exchange ideas and practices regarding all that concerns fertility and contraception. Following this ethnographic setup, even though most scholarship on religion in Israel treats these sectors as distinct groups, this ethnography includes Orthodox couples who originate from Haredi (ultra-Orthodox), Dati (Religious Zionists), and Hardal (national-Haredi) communities. However, Hasidic sects were not incorporated into this study because they usually attend their own communal-based gatherings and did not attend these nonsectorial venues.[102]

These conferences were also where I met many of my participants, especially at the beginning of this research. I owe particular gratitude to Penina, a clever Hasidic woman whom I met at one of these gatherings. Penina not only became a friend and informant but also paved the way for many other people to share their stories with me. Penina approached me when I entered the hall to attend an evening devoted to Haredi family life. She glanced at my name tag and asked: "Are you the one who wrote the paper on modesty? You must come to my talk!" I was very surprised (and a bit worried) as I followed her into the large room where she was about to speak. I found out that Penina is a Bais Yaakov seminary teacher, and her talk presented a survey of the academic research on modesty, which, according to her, was completing wrong! As I prepared for a silent getaway before I got eggs thrown at me, she began to present my own work and said, "This work is different, she gets us!" She then pointed her finger at me and said: "She is here in the room, looking for people to participate in her next study. Go talk to her!"

Anthropologists always have to find creative ways to overcome gatekeeping. I was lucky for Penina's kind invitation, that evening and beyond. With her help, as well as the help of other acquaintances (and the ever-useful snowball method), I conducted fifty interviews with a range of differently positioned social actors, from Orthodox men and women to bridal counselors, Jewish law consultants, rabbinic experts, and gynecologists. This allowed me to gain to insights from different perspectives—personal, medical, and rabbinic.

In order to gain access to personal accounts of Orthodox men, many of the interviews I conducted were couple interviews. As in other communities where intimacy and sexuality are heavily guarded, being married was a critical advantage, as "virgin ears would probably have been protected."[103] The fact that birth control is considered taboo actually worked to my advantage, as the couples were more amenable to sharing their safeguarded stories with someone they would never encounter again.

My methodological approach explicitly focused on couple interviews to showcase the dilemmas that emerge between couples throughout the book, highlighting the gendered shape of desire. Using a methodology of couple interviews, I give voice to male desires and dilemmas around Orthodox family-making to challenge hegemonic representations of Jewish masculinity and advance the social study of reproduction, where women's experiences are disproportionately centered. Even though it is ideal to interview spouses separately to minimize their influence on each other and allow disagreements to be aired safely, in this study couples were given the choice to interview either together or separately, depending on where they thought they would feel more comfortable. This was of particular importance, as flexibility was needed in order to find ways for men who are unaccustomed to speaking with women, to discuss intimate issues with a female interviewer. Nevertheless, due to the strict modesty practices and gender segregation that are customary in these communities, a male interviewer was provided when preferred by interviewees. This ethnography thus offers cutting-edge methodology by arguing that we cannot continue to study reproductive choice solely through the perspectives of women. I weave these couple interviews with observational notes made at conferences and classes on Jewish sexuality and family life, and analysis of handbooks and manuals about the Jewish family.

Returning to Penina's words "She gets us!"—this comment lingered for a while, as it captured some of my own dilemmas regarding my positionality in this research. From Penina's perspective, there were two kinds of scholars—the ones who got them, and the ones who did not. In many ways, I understood what she meant. Most of the scholars of Orthodox Judaism in Israel (and beyond) are not Orthodox. Many incorporate critical readings of Orthodox life in their analysis and in their public writing, especially regarding gender and sexuality. Penina was trying to say that my work was different—which made me simultaneously happy but also worried. Why was my work perceived as different? I wondered, was this because I am an observant Jew myself? Was it because I am married? Or because I already have children of my own? Her comment touched on my reflections about my particular positionality and how this affected the questions I was asking, my encounters in the field, and the type of analysis that I put forward.

While the complexity of the Jewish ethnographer studying Jews has been heavily discussed,[104] Jewish ethnographers are still predominantly secular. I position myself in the liberal parts of Orthodox Judaism, but being an observant Jew mattered, to me and to my interlocutors. On the one hand, it made it easier for me to "get them." On the other hand, there was also a crucial difference. While to an outsider, my being a liberal Orthodox Jews puts me in the same camp, it also serves as a threat.[105]

Being a religious feminist comes with its own baggage, and I was worried I would not be able to keep my feminist critique to myself. In a paradoxical way, I was actually worried I would not "get them." I was worried I would not be able to empathize enough with their desires to have large families, and with the cracks that emerged as things became harder and harder. While I admit that I was not fully able to understand the desire to have such large families, ethnographic empathy grew as they shared their painful stories with me. Having "only" three children of my own positioned my desires and decisions in stark contrast to those of most of the people I talked to. After a while, however, I realized that while I did not always empathize with their desires, I came to understand their pain. And I think that is one of the immense gifts of ethnography.

## Book Overview

To tell the reproductive stories of Israel's Orthodox and ultra-Orthodox Jews, I have divided this book into five chapters. Chapter 1 ethnographically explores the diverse ways that Orthodox Jews reorient their family-making desires in a context where social, religious, economic, and national values are shifting. This chapter illustrates how cracks emerge in family-making dreams, while weaving an explicit thread between personal and national imaginaries of "promised lands" and the dilemmas that arise as couples fail to attain them.

Chapter 2 illustrates how Jewish men and women cultivate new ethical choreographies by actively seeking out new spaces to share their frustrations, difficulties, and challenges. As couples struggle to live up to modern parenting ideals (presented by a state perceived as secular), the creative "repro-theologies" offered by religious educators aim to reconcile competing reproductive desires in the midst of shifting modes of reproductive governance. Advancing recent calls to study the relations between anthropology and theology, I claim that repro-theologies are not merely a product of rigid principles of Jewish theology and law. While anthropology and its possible links to Christian theology have flourished in the past years, I move here beyond Protestant formations to focus on the ways in which lived experiences are sites for creating repro-theologies.

Chapter 3 analyzes the ways in which Orthodox couples use rabbinic consultation as an ethical compass in the midst of moral uncertainty. First, it delves deeply into couples' reproductive stories, while highlighting how religious consultation has emerged as a powerful praxis of ethical self-formation. Then, I show how, for many of my interlocutors, the process of consultation was more significant than rote submission to religious rulings. As we will see, some couples "shop around" until they find a ruling that is to their liking. Some seek to fully accept and submit to religious rulings, while delegating their weighty decisions to rabbis. Others seek the authority of religious figures yet negotiate the outcomes, either embracing or rejecting rulings while taking their own preferences into account. Departing from classic debates regarding how religious leaders struggle to legitimate their authority in the eyes of their communities, I turn the lens of anthropological inquiry to the ways in which religious members engage with authorities in their everyday lives. I argue that the analysis of engagement with religious authorities requires attention to inner diversity and the wide range of interpretations and practices within Orthodoxy.

What types of decisions are made amid changing political and economic infrastructures? Chapter 4 illustrates how contemporary religious reproduction requires new reproductive decision-making frameworks. I explore how Orthodox couples engage in contraception while blurring the categories of choice, desire, and intentionality. As uncertainty and ambivalence prevail, reproductive decision-making entails elements of adaptability that create (almost) inconceivable situations in which children born to parents using birth control are still wanted. Unraveling the illusion of a binary model of planned/unplanned parenthood, I show how couples chose to postpone and welcome pregnancies at the same time.

Chapter 5 illustrates how religious elites rethink reproductive obligations, illustrating how religious critique is based on particular social and cultural capital. Following Shellee Colen's term "stratified reproduction,"[106] I demonstrate how these strategies create hidden power relations by which some people are empowered to nurture and reproduce, while others are disempowered. Secrecy creates a distinction between different subgroups of Orthodox communities, as it is specifically the newcomers, the *baalei teshuva* (returnees), who are currently carrying most of the fertility load. This phenomenon obliges us to rethink the ideological and harmonious picture of religious life by focusing on religious capital and power in the context of stratified reproduction.

The coda takes the reader back to a macroanalysis of Israel's reproductive governance today. In the aftermath of thorny state-religion tensions amid the COVID-19 pandemic and recent shifts in Israeli politics, this section of the book points to new developments in the current state of reproductive politics. I highlight how a new set of desires drive Israel's agenda today as there has been a shift from a desire to reproduce Jews to a desire to maintain a Jewish majority of a particular kind. Accordingly, the coda stresses the importance of studying desire ethnographically while offering an ethnographic tool kit and language with which to do so.

My interest in religious family-making desires in Israel amid shifting forms of reproductive governance stems from my experiences as an anthropologist and a mother. I was born in the United States but grew up in Israel amid this social transformation, where my husband and I brought up our three children. Amid this social change, my own embodied experience led to the intellectual questions that I explore in this book,[107] namely, what and who constructs our most basic desires; how gender, religious ideals, and state policy shape the most intimate family dreams and desires; and how biomedical technologies, bodies, and Orthodox cosmologies bring forward particular modes of ethical decision-making during particular moments in history. My hope is that paying close attention to this particular moment in the reproductive governance of Orthodox Jews in Israel will provoke conversations about the delicate balance between personal desire and the state, an ethical choreography that lives at the heart of the human condition all over the globe.

# 1

# Cracks

It is a cold Saturday night in mid-December. I enter a somewhat rundown theater hall to watch *Vatahar Vateled* ("And she conceived and gave birth"), a new solo performance by a religious woman named Rachel Keshet. I take my seat in the small theater, huddling together with a crowd of roughly fifty women on brown wooden benches. A spotlight highlights the figure of a woman standing at the center of the stage, dressed in a tight yellow dress. Even though the three-quarter-length sleeves and floor-length dress reflect a modest choice, the dress is very tight, emphasizing every curve of her body and accentuating the marks remaining from her seven pregnancies.

She stares at the crowd and begins to speak monotonously: "I wake up in the morning and wash my face. Look into the mirror with the green frame. I brush my teeth with my purple toothbrush. I make the sandwiches. Spread the cottage cheese. Take off the crust. Cut up the cucumbers. Put them in a box. Wake them up, get them dressed, brush their hair. I hug, then discipline, and push them out the door." She repeats her description of her morning routine over and over, while increasing the speed with each repetition. She then begins to incorporate biblical verses into her daily to-do list. I can make out the verse from Genesis (18:6): "And Abraham hastened into the tent unto Sarah, and said: 'Make ready quickly three measures of fine meal, knead it, and make cakes.'"

Keshet begins to walk around the stage, and I realize that her hair is connected to the ceiling with a set of strings. As she moves around the empty stage, her hair constantly drags behind her. Divided into four parts, each of which is attached to a string, her hair is pulled by her every movement, either tightening or unravelling, depending on the direction she walks. I refocus my attention on her words and realize she is reciting the biblical birth stories of the Jewish matriarchs. As she retells these stories, she offers her own interpretations through intonations and rhythm. She repeats the biblical verse "And she conceived and she gave birth." With each iteration, she squats down and pretends to be in labor. She repeats these verses, again and again, as she screams out in agony, as if she is giving birth right there on the stage. "And she conceived and she gave birth." I wonder how it feels to replicate the story of Rachel, her namesake, who dies during childbirth. As she squats down lower and lower, she pulls the string so hard, I am worried it might rip. It looks painful. She is unable to move as far as she wants. She is confined by her hair.

\* \* \*

As I watched Rachel Keshet's performance, I realized that this was a visual representation of the constant pain I heard while couples shared their family-building stories with me.[1] As the woman sitting next to me remarked as the show concluded: "I feel like she is telling my story." Keshet's constant reference to and critical reading of biblical reproduction highlight the painful cracks that appear in family-making ideals of religious women and men, which depart from the expectations with which they were raised. I view the strings that confound her as visual metaphors for the parts of her life that constrain her. She is caught, literally, between heaven and earth, between age-old prenatal ideals and the everyday life hardships they entail.

At times during the play I could see that the string also serves as a central axis in her life, offering stability as she conducts her everyday duties. But as she squats down, again and again, she demonstrates how each birth entails an existential pull, threatening to rupture the string, which might rip, right in front of our eyes. Sitting in the crowd that evening, I realized that Keshet was begging us to pay attention to the real hardships entailed in making a large family. While she draws on religious ideals in the play, her visual performance offers a new soundtrack to these biblical narratives. She asks us to look beyond these monotonous descriptions of childbirth while paying attention to the cracks that emerge with the birth of each child.

This chapter exposes the deep family frustrations couples shared with me during my fieldwork. By paying careful attention to these frustrations, I go beyond the tendency to attribute religious ideas about reproduction to biblical imagery to "be fruitful and multiply," which obscures the painful cracks that appear in family-making. As noted earlier, I call these ambivalences "cracks" to highlight the painful gaps I found between large-family ideals and lived realities. Building on Keshet's creative use of a string on the verge of ripping, I introduce the variety of challenges couples shared with me, which threatened to rip the fabric that holds their lives together. In particular, I focus on two types of frustration that were common among the men and women I met yet rarely surface in ideological-heavy depictions of Orthodox reproduction: economic concerns and bodily strains. I situate these frustrations in a particular context where religious, economic, and national values are shifting amid an inadequate infrastructure of sex education among Orthodox Jews.[2]

While sex education in other contexts typically focuses on bodily development, sex, sexuality, consent, and relationships, Jewish premarriage classes primarily focus on the halachic aspects of Jewish marriage.[3] The "laws of purity," often called *taharat hamishpacha*, are an elaborate menstruation defilement and purification system that organizes marital sexuality through a recurring cycle of purity and impurity.[4] These laws are taught as part of a series of one-on-one classes that range in length and price (typically four to ten hourly meetings at around 100 shekels per class for women, while men, if they go at all, will have one or two free meetings with a rabbi). These classes vary in their quality, quantity, and philosophy (which are dependent on the particular teacher). While most focus on knowledge transmission of the laws of purity, an array of topics may be covered, from emotional to psychological, and limited sexual education. Informal chats about forbidden subjects likely exist, but formal sex education was often referred

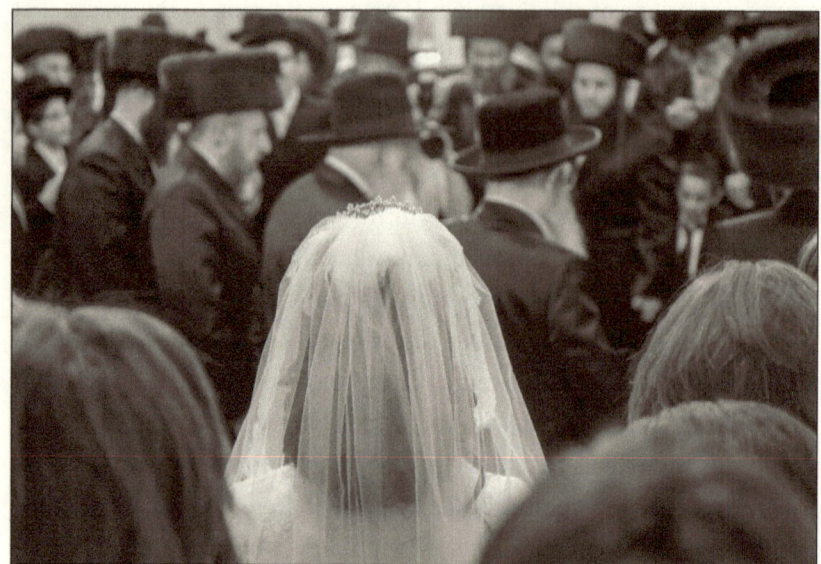

FIGURE 1.1. Jewish wedding ceremony. Photo by Avishag Shaar-Yashuv.

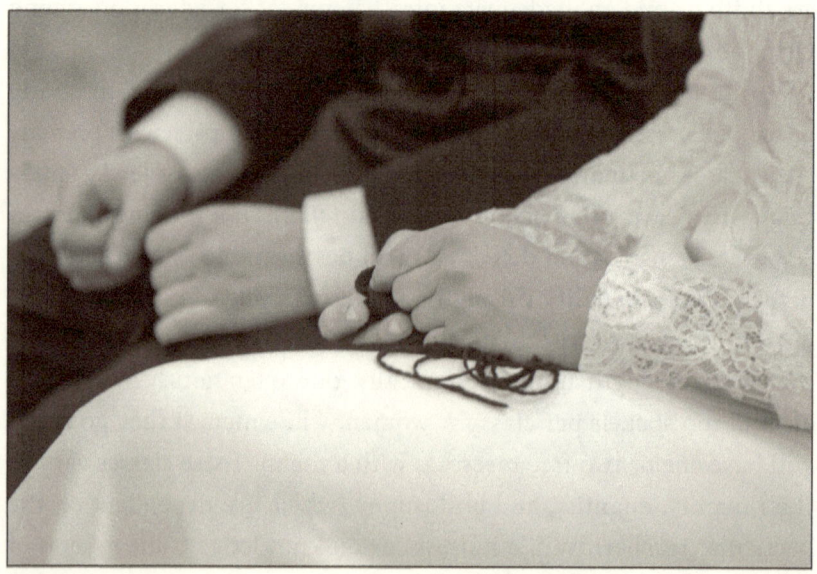

FIGURE 1.2. Bride and groom. Photo by Avishag Shaar-Yashuv.

to briefly, usually as part of the last session; couples perceived these classes as simple introductions to bodily education but then searched for secondary avenues to learn more about sexuality, marital relations, and the realities of reproductive lives.[5]

Because sex education is scarce, couples' debates about contraception are punctuated by limited knowledge regarding permissible birth control techniques. While most bridal teachers will suggest an appointment with a gynecologist to make sure the bride-to-be's cycle does not coincide with the wedding (a situation that is called *chuppat niddah*), they typically use this topic to promote procreation, which brides are expected to realize quickly, within a year of marriage. As a consequence, even though they spent weeks preparing for marriage, most women will enter the first phase of their sexual and reproductive life with almost no knowledge about contraception. These circumstances create a particular configuration of reproductive decision-making that only begins after couples are married and sexually active, typically after they are already concerned with the care of a few children.

In focusing on the ways in which economic concerns figured into couples' narratives, even though economic concerns have traditionally been viewed as a "bad" and "secular" reason to prevent pregnancies, we can see how these economic logics slowly emerge within couples' narratives while also charting the ethical choreographies these new frameworks entail. Building on Sarah Ahmed's work, I argue that economic concerns and bodily strains open up new horizons as couples realize they cannot follow the normative "desire lines" that orient toward a large family. By contextualizing the particular conditions in which family cracks emerge, I argue that pronatal ideals do not merely replicate age-old dogmas but are shaped (and reshaped) by shifting state policies. While highlighting moments of doubt is a common challenge in ethnographic research,[6] showcasing cracks in the context of Orthodox family-making is especially telling as Orthodox men and women are often depicted as blindly committed to procreation.

## Banks and Blessings

I watch as Chava runs to catch her bus to Ofakim, a small and developing city in southern Israel. I see her clutch a brown purse close to her body as she disappears into the busy crowd of people moving toward the central bus station. I had just met Chava at a café in Jerusalem. Chava, a Haredi graphic designer, was working hard to establish herself in the field. Her husband, Yaakov, wanted to study Torah full-time but had recently begun teaching in a primary school because they were having trouble making ends meet. They had three children, and Chava was not sure they could handle another one. "I am not sure what to do," she shared with me. When I asked her about contraception, she recalled her struggles: "I have had bad experiences with pills. They gave me terrible headaches, but what else can I do? I don't want to insert an IUD. It seems crazy to go through such a process.... I will want to have another child soon."

Chava's account offers a glimpse into a particular configuration of reproductive decision-making that only began after she was married and sexually active. As noted earlier, within the Orthodox community, sexuality is addressed in hushed tones, and family planning is not formally broached until marriage preparation, and often only afterward. These communal norms are the circumstances within which Chava began to negotiate contraception, in the context of the hardships of everyday life and care for her three children. These circumstances also frame some types of contraception, like an IUD, as irrelevant for someone who wants a break but is also planning on having more children relatively soon. Similar to Chava, other women with whom I spoke also often referred to IUDs as an intrusive intervention. In addition, after an IUD is inserted, women usually experience a few months of spotting. While this may seem like an unpleasant but unimportant side effect, for a religious woman it means a few months when she may not be able to even touch her husband, which added to couples' reluctance.

One of the things that struck me about Chava's story is that even though she grapples with these questions, she continued to stall her decision-making. With a frustrated shrug, she said: "Somehow, I keep on forgetting about it. I am so busy. By the time the day is over I am so tired, I don't have the strength to think about it. . . . And then mikvah [ritual bath] night comes and I don't know what to do. . . . Maybe it has been enough time already and I should just prepare to have another child. But, I also need to put effort into my job. As a freelancer, it is really hard. I just don't know. I don't know."

Chava's questions still ring in my ear; I still do not know what she decided to do. Even though she admitted that she loses sleep over this question, she continually defers her decisions until the monthly reminder arrives—mikvah night. In accordance with Jewish *niddah* (menstrual) laws, during menstruation, sexual intercourse is prohibited between married couples until the woman has immersed herself in a ritual bath, which conveniently falls on the part of the month when women are most fertile.

Chava's indecisiveness was shared by many others. While many men and women dreamed about being parents from a young age, they found their high-fertility dreams hard to achieve in real life. Despite the importance of reproduction, economic strains and cultural changes regarding parenting ideals, gender, body, and work-family balance constitute a real challenge. Couples like Chava and her husband describe their struggles in personal terms, but their concerns are deeply linked to, and embedded in, structural, cultural, and economic changes introduced in 2003, noted earlier, which create cracks in the idealized dream of the large Jewish family.

Poverty is a deep-seated challenge for Israel's Haredi families. In 2016, the National Insurance Institute in Israel released a report indicating that 45.1 percent of Haredi families are under the poverty line. This is much greater than the general rate of poverty in Israel, which was 18.5 percent in 2016.[7] After years of steady government child support, most large families have been especially vulnerable to the deep cutbacks in Israel's child allowance since 2003.[8] Until 2003, a family with ten children received roughly 6,000 New Israeli Shekels (NIS) from the Israeli government. Since 2003, that same family might only receive between 2,000 and 3,000 NIS, leaving them to meet the costs of inflation without additional support.

These cutbacks have forced couples to move out of geographically central, religious neighborhoods, such as those in Jerusalem, to more peripheral, smaller communities and settlements, like Ofakim, where Chava and her family reside. Even though most Haredi women work outside their homes, these economic changes have caused many women to delay the timing of their marriage and search for higher-paid work.[9] These developments have also hindered the Haredi man's ability to devote himself fully to Torah study, which is also clearly visible in Yaakov's choice to begin to teach in an elementary school. Yaakov is not unique in this way. The ascetic yeshiva-based ideology (which, as noted previously, is a much more recent phenomenon than typically described) has become an onerous burden on the average household for many. These economic hardships, along with the realization that a considerable percentage of male adults simply lack the temperament or motivation for full-time study, have stoked intracommunal tensions and are even prompting far-reaching changes.[10]

And, still, among most Orthodox communities, economic concerns were perceived as "problematic." As Hannah, a national-Haredi educator said to a room filled with Orthodox mothers in one of the family conferences I attended: "What, are we like the secular Jews who don't have a fourth child because they would need to get a new car?" Even though this rhetoric runs deep in Orthodox frameworks, everyday economic struggles pushed the men and women I met to cultivate new desires as they learned to bring economic calculations into their family decision-making process. As I entered the homes of married couples, I got used to sitting on couches with torn covers, dining room tables with missing chairs, and bedrooms with two or three sets of rickety bunk beds. I saw how mothers prepared meals carefully, buying food in bulk, using bread crusts to make croutons, and shopping at the end of the day to get cheaper prices.

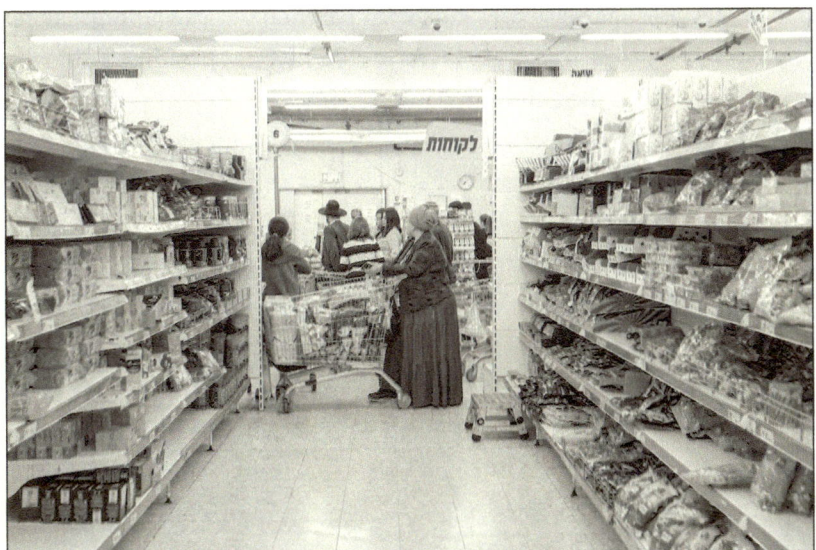

FIGURE 1.3. Supermarket in Jerusalem. Photo by Avishag Shaar-Yashuv.

I also encountered couples who were not struggling financially but who also seemed to experience difficulties as their struggles were deeply linked to "Western" ideals of "intensive parenting," a form of parenting standards that are not achievable for large families.[11] As Deborah Golden, Lauren Erdreich, and Sveta Robermen show,[12] non-Haredi Jewish parents in Israel, and especially mothers, have been heavily influenced by a model of intensive parenting that urges parents to spend a tremendous amount of time, energy, and money on raising their children.[13] These methods for "appropriate" child-rearing are not only child-centered, emotionally consuming, and labor-intensive but also expensive. In households with large families, parents often divide household labor and childcare among older siblings, who take on many responsibilities, preparing food, bringing their younger siblings to childcare, and often helping with other tasks such as homework. Parents often do not have the time or money for extracurricular activities and other middle-class parental responsibilities. As intensive parenting norms challenge their realities, parents I met often stated that they felt bad about tasking their older kids with parental duties and not having enough money to *lehashkia* (to invest and be invested), both emotionally and financially, in the children.

In her work on Agudat Efrat, Israel's most prominent nonprofit anti-abortion group, Michal Raucher shows how generous financial aid is provided to pregnant women who are considering abortions but are persuaded to continue their pregnancies despite dire financial circumstances. Guided by a post-Holocaust and Zionist ideology, Agudat Efrat's objective is to increase the Jewish population by making sure children are not aborted for "unnecessary reasons." But Agudat Efrat also receives frequent requests for assistance from women who have already given birth to children they are unable to support. Even though the explicit organizational mission is to support women who are considering abortion, it does offer support to Haredi women, even after they have already given birth. In this sense, their work is similar to that of other Jewish free loan funds (*gemachs*) that support Haredi men and women in various aspects of their financial needs.[14] These community-based charities offer a web of support—from diapers to strollers to clothing—to families who struggle economically for the entirety of their lives.

While financial challenges create ruptures in the ability to actualize high-fertility needs, financial stress is also linked to questions of career and work-life balance as well as to personal growth and leisure ideals.[15] Furthermore, as gender ideals and practices transform, men and women express discontent with their one-dimensional gender roles, and some are even clamoring openly for reform.[16]

In her book *Yeshiva Fundamentalism*, Nurit Stadler demonstrates how modern psychological trends have contributed to the rise of a new ideal of the Haredi father. She describes how a "discourse of domestication" initiated a movement that encourages Haredi men to return to their families. Following Stadler's work, recent studies show that Haredi fathers are taking on more and more family responsibilities.[17] For example, the yeshivot have a built-in afternoon break, which has created a perfect opportunity for Haredi fathers to chip in by picking their children up from school or preparing lunch for the children when they come home. Yet, this pragmatic innovation creates ambivalence among many Haredi men because this care work challenges the ideal of full devotion to Torah study. Stadler describes how some Haredi fathers overcome this ambivalence by creating a "domestication of piety," which allows them to bring the "spirit of the yeshiva home" by becoming more involved in child education and offering emotional support, which is still perceived as "feminine work."

Yet, even though they might publicly downplay their involvement in housework and childcare in the face of social pressure, the Haredi men I spoke with voiced a desire to play an even more prominent role in parenting. As Menachem, a Haredi father, put it: "I love being with my children. This might sound a bit unconventional, but I don't think this needs to be only a job for women. I also want to be a father. And, I don't mean that I want to help with my children. What am I a babysitter? I can't babysit my own children! They are my responsibility to begin with!" As their fatherhood desires develop, Haredi men often also critique their own upbringing, which entails a painful understanding that perhaps their fathers should or could have been a more meaningful part of their childhood.

As they questioned these gendered ideals in the context of the family unit, couples debated the traditional gender division of household labor and parenting and also critiqued ideals of romance. As these ideals shift, couples struggle to find suitable models for Orthodox romance. Shlomo, whose story appeared in the introduction, explained painfully how he and his wife, Miriam, "never really had time to build our own relationship." Large families take a toll on family life, pushing both men and women to reorient their ways. In line with these new desires, romance often seemed to be an extremely painful topic. As couples tended to marry quickly (usually with very little physical involvement beforehand) and have a child within twelve months, they did not have much time to be just a couple. Exacerbated by a dearth of religious ideals of romance due to issues of modesty, Orthodox couples searched for appropriate ways to be intimate.[18] As Meir, one of the Haredi fathers, shared with me: "I had a wonderful idea of how to be a caring father, but I had no idea how to be a spouse. I never saw my parents in that way."

## Pregnant Is Beautiful?

Yossi is a Haredi man in his late thirties who spent most of his time studying in yeshiva. Over the past few years, he had also been studying for a bachelor's degree at the Open University to eventually find a way to support his family. Although his wife works as a kindergarten teacher, they are still struggling financially. Yossi was working hard to keep up with his academic requirements, which included English and math, topics he barely studied while growing up.[19] I met him for coffee next to the library at Hebrew University's Givat Ram campus, where he often came to use the computers because he did not want to bring a laptop into his home. Yossi smiled when he talked about his wife and three children. As the conversation went deeper, he recalled what his mother went through to have nine children:

> My mother spent so much time in the hospital each time she was pregnant. As the oldest son in a family with nine kids, I could see how hard it was on her body. I knew that having children was very important to her, but it was very hard for me too. When I grew up I promised myself that I would never let that happen to my wife. Having lots of children should not come at the price of one's health!

As Yossi's narrative highlights the bodily pains his mother went through, I realized how atypical this explicit critique was. While most of the couples I spoke to referred to the heavy toll multiple pregnancies have on the female body, they typically attempted to overcome that challenge unless the woman had a severe medical condition. Women often complained about how consecutive births weakened their pelvises and left their bodies with stretch marks and bulging varicose veins, yet it was hard to admit that these bodily challenges could become a factor in their decision-making. In fact, in many of the marriage guidebooks women commonly read, they were continuously persuaded to accept the shifting forms of their bodies as part of their fertility "mission."

In her popular book *A Woman's Life*, Dr. Chana Katan, a religious gynecologist and mother of thirteen who is well known for promoting large families, writes:

> There are some women who are embarrassed by their constantly pregnant look, even though it is the most beautiful look there is; that is why every time a first-time pregnant woman comes to my clinic, I give her a "pregnancy kit" that I prepared (including a list of instructions, tests, and explanations, etc.) and also Yitzchak Shalev's poem "A Pregnancy Dress," a poem I received from my mother-in-law when I was pregnant for the first time.[20]

"A Pregnancy Dress" is a popular Hebrew poem, written from the perspective of a husband who watches his wife struggle with her pregnant appearance. In one of the verses he comments: "You will never know how beautiful you looked in those days when we were guessing whether it would be a boy or a girl." Offering this poem to a young woman on her first visit to a gynecologist captures how boundaries between the medical, the ethical, and the aesthetic are blurred in the Israeli repro-context. Amid this prevalent rhetoric, women are taught to adopt the "pregnant is beautiful" perspective, which makes it hard for them to admit they struggle with the marks multiple pregnancies leave on their bodies.

Dr. Katan also offers idealized depictions of pain throughout her popular books. For example, she tells the story of a twenty-two-year-old mother of three who described how her varicose veins bulge and hurt, yet the woman describes her pains as follows: "I do not complain, these are not just varicose veins on my legs, I call them pictures from my future children!"[21] Here, too, Dr. Katan uses this creative narrative to discipline women to rethink their bodily pain and aesthetics.[22] They are taught to perceive these pains as a necessary step to bring forward more children.

The intensity of this reproductive disciplining was vividly clear to me during one of the bridal training classes I attended. Together with a group of roughly forty women, I participated in a series of weekly classes as part of a yearlong training to become a bridal teacher. While most of the classes focused on issues in Jewish law and spiritual preparation for marriage, a few classes focused on physiology. In one of them, a physical therapist arrived to discuss the importance of bodily awareness. As necessary background, she told the participants her own story of how she became an expert on postnatal support:

> I got married late and wanted to have a large family, so I had three children, one after another, without waiting at all. After my third pregnancy, I went to the bathroom and could see something sticking out. . . . I went to the doctor, who told me I must fix this before I have any more children. He referred me to a French woman who just immigrated to Israel and had a new approach to strengthening pelvic muscles. I went to see her, and she promised to help me. She agreed that I must take a break before I can have more children. But I really wanted more, so we worked hard. And, thank God! It didn't get any worse! Well, it didn't go exactly back to normal, but it didn't get any worse. Thank God, I have had four more children this way, and I am grateful!

I watched the other women in the room as she told this story. Everyone was so happy for her. They congratulated her and asked for her phone number to share with their friends. Even though she was invited to speak about bodily awareness, the physical therapist did not refer to this condition—likely a prolapsed uterus—to raise awareness that it is an issue that needs more attention. She mentioned that they worked to strengthen her pelvic muscles, but instead of using this instance to educate on the importance of seeking more medical attention, her focus remained on having large families. I wondered whether anyone thought to ask her what the bodily limits are and whether there are physical conditions that require a respite from pregnancies.

Although none of the women asked these questions publicly, I found couples who were taking bodily concerns into their decision-making. The ambivalence around the body really struck home when I spoke to Liat after the birth of her third child. She told me:

> After a few months, I realized that my pelvic muscles had been stretched to the point that I had occasional leaking urine. I found that if I laughed out loud or wanted to dance at a wedding, this would likely come at a cost. I couldn't believe this was the consequence of having three children one after another. No one had prepared me for this. I went to the doctor, who seemed surprised that I wasn't doing Kegel exercises daily. I had never heard of this beforehand, not from my own doctor nor from my bridal teacher. I wasn't sure what to do. I wanted to have more children, but I also thought perhaps I shouldn't have any more children until I would be able to laugh without worrying about controlling my urine. On the other hand, I wonder—is this really a good enough reason to wait?

For Liat, a stance that involved taking her body into account emerged only after the birth of her third child. As she pondered contraception, she critiqued her medical and religious systems for not preparing her for the potential tolls consecutive birthing would have on her body. And, still, Liat is not sure whether this is a "good enough" reason to put off having more children.

Indeed, one of the main things that struck me while hearing couples' fertility narratives was how long couples debated this topic. For most of the couples I met, choosing a spouse was probably the biggest life decision they made, and children were a natural outcome. They never really asked themselves whether or not they wanted to become parents. Thus, most couples started to question these high fertility norms only after they became parents. Moreover, it was not easy to realize that "they need a break," as many of my interviewees put it. Similar to findings of other anthropologists, this realization was understood as a failure to succeed in one of the most basic and important roles in life, particularly for women whose fertility performance is critical to their social status.²³

## Pick Your Poison

When I got engaged to be married, I was in middle of fieldwork in a Bais Yaakov seminary, and a few of the teachers, as well as other religious educators from other denominations, offered to help me prepare for my upcoming wedding. As a young anthropologist, I was quite excited by these offers, which allowed a rare autoethnographic exploration of bridal preparation, so I said yes—to everyone. Each class I attended was taught by a different teacher from a particular stream of Orthodox Judaism, offering a unique vantage point to compare different views on contraception.

I was not surprised when each teacher recommended I purchase a different guidebook. My Haredi bridal teacher suggested *Teharat Bat Yisrael* (*The Purity of the Daughter of Israel*), written by Rabbi Kalman Kehana, and my modern-Orthodox mentor recommended *Ish Veisha* (*Man and Woman*), written by Rabbi Elyashiv Khnol. I also purchased *Netivot Tohar* (*Paths of Purity*), a book that is usually offered to Sephardi brides, as well as to *baalei teshuva* (returnees).

While I found many differences among these guidebooks, their attitudes toward contraception were strikingly similar: all books discussed contraception briefly at the end of the book. For example, *Teharat Bat Yisrael* has nineteen chapters. The final chapter, entitled "The Prohibition to Prevent Pregnancies," offers one rather straightforward paragraph:

> Prevention of pregnancy, in any way, is one of the most severe prohibitions. A husband and wife should be very careful not to fail in such a serious sin. Even if the doctors say that there is a life concern in case of a pregnancy, the couple should not decide themselves, but rather ask a wise scholar.²⁴

The other two marriage guidebooks I have mentioned offer a slightly more detailed discussion, but both of them state the importance of building a large family and recommend consulting a rabbi when considering contraception. They also state that when contraception is allowed (or even obligated for medical reasons), the Pill was a preferred method among most Orthodox rabbis, whereas mechanical methods like the condom, if allowed at all, are least preferred.

These stringent views, as promulgated within these Orthodox communities, run contrary to the detailed debates about contraception in Jewish law, which do take other considerations into account. In fact, in the Talmud the religious obligation to procreate specifies only one or two children.[25] As Ronit Irshai has shown,[26] within the debate about procreation and family planning there is also an entire system of individual concerns that may be taken into consideration, such as physical and mental health, financial issues, and child welfare, to name a few.[27] Yet, these detailed accounts rarely appear in the marriage guidebooks I collected (leading, as we will see, to an obscure system of stratified knowledge).

I found that even when bridal teachers decide to explicitly discuss contraception, they tend to portray it as *bedieved*, a concept in Jewish law that means it is only allowed ex post facto, when no other options are available. As Ruchi, one of bridal teachers told me:

> It is really important for me to tell brides what contraception exists. I have realized that many brides have no idea what is out there, and it is my responsibility to make sure they know. So, I go through all the different kinds of contraception—making sure they understand the pros and cons of each one, and then I say: you can pick your poison.

Ruchi's narrative offers a striking paradox. Even though she feels that it is her responsibility to provide brides with a basic understanding of contraception, she frames contraceptive use as "poison." Thus, while she is offering important contraception knowledge, she is also perpetuating a narrative that vilifies contraception, which should only be used when there is no other choice.

Even after deciding to pursue using birth control, many couples complained about the limited options available. As Rivka, a modern-Orthodox woman from a small village in northern Israel, shared with me:

> I started taking the Pill and suffered from terrible headaches. I went back to the doctor, and she suggested an IUD. That seemed like too much. I went home and didn't know what to do. Mikvah night was approaching.... I spoke to my husband, and he said that I should go to the mikvah. We would touch without... you know.... I am lucky to be married to such a gentle and understanding man. We were like this for six months. I just couldn't do it.

Rivka explained how she and her husband refrained from sex for six months because she could not find suitable contraception. Other couples I met tried sponges or various spermicides, and some even used condoms although they were considered nonpermissible. Even though many secular women in Israel use IUDs,[28] religious women, like Rivka, were hesitant to use them. As noted earlier, many women perceived an IUD as too intrusive. Also, as previously mentioned, due to the spotting side effects that are common after insertion of an IUD, couples were reluctant to engage in contraception that would entail entire months when they might not be able to touch. Hence, I found that IUDs were typically used when a couple had decided to stop having children or made a conscious decision to wait for a few years before having the next child, which was quite uncommon.

This meant that most women relied on hormonal pills, which left women like Rivka searching for creative alternatives when hormones were not a viable option for them. Among these women, the diaphragm became a relevant solution. While, in the past, the permissibility of a diaphragm has been contested, its growing use has deemed it "kosher" according to many rabbinic leaders. As they searched for the best contraception for them, women would share how happy they were when their period arrived and how restless they would get when their periods were late. Some succeeded in preventing pregnancies, but babies were still conceived as couples learned how to use a diaphragm for the first time or used one without having it properly fitted. Sometimes, couples were still deliberating whether they should use contraception but continued to have children as their uncertainty and limited knowledge merged. Sometimes, as hard as it was for them to admit, this baby may have been one child too much.

Reorienting Desire

Why were these decisions so hard to make? Having a large family was not only a communal norm but also a personal desire. In fact, it was a desire that was hard to let go. For the couples I spoke with, confronting the ways they fall short of their parenting ideals was fused with ethical uncertainty. Even though the desire for large families was unequivocal for most of their life, the cracks they experienced unearthed the potential for other aspirations. Yet, these new desires created a deep disorientation, a life without a clear ethical object of directionality. I find Sara Ahmed's attention to queer orientation helpful to illustrate this conundrum:

> For a life to count as a good life, it must return the debt of its life by taking on the direction promised as a social good, which means imagining one's futurity in terms of reaching certain points along a life course. Such points accumulate, creating the impression of a straight line. To follow such a line might be a way to become straight, by not deviating at any point.[29]

While Ahmed uses this framework to analyze the reorientation of queer desire, I take on this analytical framework to characterize how men and women fail to live up to the communal orientation toward a "good" life.[30] The failure to desire the idealized "large Jewish family" is similar to the failure (and resistance) to follow the straight line.[31] In the context of reproduction, not being able to follow normative desire lines creates ethical uncertainty as these accumulated points that create an impression of straight "lines" are perceived as necessary to making a good life. For some of my interlocuters, their failures reflected a desire to follow the communal norm of large families, a moral commitment they would wish to continue—if only there had been better circumstances. For others, these disparities were translated into critical reflections of the "ideal" Jewish family, while questioning patriarchal divisions of labor and the traditional expectations these demands put on men and women. In other words, these cracks shattered patriarchal ideals in a context of religious Orthodoxy.

The comparison to queer deviation is also useful because it helps to highlight the complexity of reorientation in the absence of relevant models—or, to paraphrase Ahmed, the disorientation that emerges when there are no "lines" to follow/reproduce. Anthropologist Rhoda Kanaaneh has shown how Palestinian women in Israel assimilated the pressure to lower their fertility levels by reorienting their reproductive choices to align with "Western" family sizes. Yet, the couples I met did not have a clear alternative family model with which they wished to align their new desires. While changing directions provides a hope toward a better future, when we do not know where some paths will take us, the risk of "departure from the straight and the narrow, makes new futures possible, which might involve going astray, getting lost."[32] The questions that Miriam voiced in the introduction—"Who is first? My husband? My children? The house? Work? My body? Who is first?"—vividly capture this sense of confusion.

Getting lost between desires and lived realities necessitates both an individual and a collective reorientation toward "the good." For many of the men and women I met, desire lines constituted an individual desire for a large family but were also linked to imaginings for a good life on a collective level, which reflect national-religious political projects of populating the promised land. While the promised land is typically understood as a theo-political geographic concept, Ahmed's work collapses both geographic and sexual orientations into "spaces." For the men and women I met, continuing traditional desire lines meant that there is also a redemptive promise lingering in the future. As cracks in their family dreams shatter their individual and communal desires, temporal ideals of promise are also jeopardized.

Amid this ethical uncertainty, Orthodox men and women learn to perform a new ethical choreography, a concept I borrow from Charis Thompson and rework to demonstrate the dynamics by which technical, scientific, gender, legal, political, financial, and theological sensitivities are coordinated to make an ethical life. The next chapter illustrates the first steps couples take in this ethical choreography, as they partake in various sex education and family education classes in search of new ethical compasses.

2

# Repro-Theologies in the Promised Land

"What a diverse group of mothers!" I wrote sarcastically in my notes, after attending an evening class dedicated to parenting in late December. The panelists that night—a mother of seven from Ramat Gan, a mother of ten from Jerusalem, and a mother of fourteen from the settlement of Eli—each shared their personal tips for parenting large families. As the chair of the panel (who shared with the crowd that she struggles with six children of her own) solicited questions from the audience, a young mother wearing a colorful headscarf who was sitting in the back of the room raised her hand. After the microphone was passed to her, she began to speak: "I appreciate the tips that you are all offering, but I am just so exhausted. You have focused on what we can do to help our children, but what about us? What tips do you have for me? How do I find the strength to continue?"

The panelists each offered what they perceived as theological and practical ways to "find strength." However, the young mother's question stayed with me. As I attended different classes and courses devoted to the Jewish family, I realized that her request helped to explain the issue that was eating away at me while I attended these classes: What motivates such busy parents to leave their homes, find (and pay for) a babysitter, and devote an entire evening or day to this topic? I found that as large-family dreams come up against the difficulties of lived reality, one of the main steps Jewish men and women take as they cultivate new ethical choreographies is actively seeking out new spaces in which to share their frustrations, difficulties, and challenges.

Over the past twenty years, there has been immense growth in adult education courses, classes, and lectures dedicated to the "Jewish family." These classes are specifically tailored to the changing needs of religious

Jews, but some offer ways to combat daily challenges while continuing the quest for large families, whereas others use these spaces to assist couples as they reorient their desires away from the large-family dream. At the heart of many of these events is a mission to educate Jewish men and women while offering tools to help them navigate the challenges that come with the tough realities of family life in contemporary Israel. Most of these efforts are founded on the belief that marriage success is a product of individual skills and couples' dynamics, and that families can acquire specific skills (both emotional and managerial) to enable them to pursue the quest for large families. These ideas are informed by a burgeoning growth in the number of Jewish relationship coaches, psychologists, sex therapists, and medical experts who posit that having a healthy family is something that one can learn how to do, and that people who receive the appropriate information can develop the attributed skills necessary to continue idealized notions of the Jewish family.

While much literature on Jewish reproduction in Israel offers an ideological picture of religious reproduction, I found that educators rarely inspired Orthodox couples to continue the quest for large families through post-Holocaust and Zionist ideals as they have done before.[1] Instead, educators put forward more individualistic sources of inspiration that offer creative ways to combat the real "wars" couples are currently fighting: exhaustion, nausea, and the desire to devote energy to building intimate relationships with their spouses. Some educators, though, take the growing social and economic structural constraints more seriously. Taking a more systematic look at the hardships with which couples are currently grappling, these educators create instructive spaces to assist couples as they reorient their desires and offer alternatives to the exclusive model of large families.

Whether challenging or reinforcing the idea of having large families, educators fuse practical, emotional, and theological notions into what I call "repro-theologies" to highlight the creative (and procreative) ways lived experience brings forward new theological insight.[2] Scholars of reproduction tend to draw their understandings of particular "theologies" about reproduction from canonical religious texts,[3] whether those of Judaism, Islam, Christianity, or non-Abrahamic traditions such as Buddhism or Hinduism. These accounts often focus on theological questions, such as human-divine relations, religious law, and religious authority.[4] But theology is not only about "the God question," or about negotiating canonical texts. By referring to lay attitudes toward family-making as "repro-theologies," my analysis accounts for theologies that emerge from the lived experiences of both men and women. Advancing recent calls to study the relations between anthropology and theology,[5] I claim that repro-theologies are not merely a product of rigid principles of Jewish theology and law. While theoretical links between anthropology and Christian theology have flourished in the past years, I move here beyond Protestant formations to focus on the ways in which lived experiences are sites for creating repro-theologies.[6] In her book *The Obligated Self*, feminist Jewish studies scholar Mara Benjamin argues that engaging with real life can enhance "our ability to engage the theological and ethical significance of the world we inhabit."[7] In a similar vein, as the telos of large families is threatened, repro-theologies are formed by the lived experiences of men and women who offer theological insights to concepts such as religious obligation and its limits.

Based on my observations at more than forty family education events, I chronicle moments of insight and analysis of these moral dimensions of family-making. Further, I consider the dynamics and coherence, as well as the divergences, between the events, the individuals, and the organizations that arrange them. In what follows, I sketch the landscape of Jewish family education at the time of my fieldwork, taking into account that this landscape constantly changes. For example, the emergence of COVID-19 posed particular challenges to Jewish parents, who continued to debate about having more children as the typical boundaries between work and family and their support structures evaporated into thin air. I show how competing fertility ideals and parenting norms are at play in different education programs. While many educators aim to reconcile between competing desires by offering practical strategies to continue the quest for large families, other religious educators reinterpret Jewish reproduction through creative approaches to religious texts, as well as critical constructions of contemporary parenting ideals, gender, work-family balance, and beauty.

## Sketching the Landscape of Jewish Family Education

It is a hot Tuesday morning as I search for a place to park in the parking lot of Binyanei Hauma, a convention center located in the center of Jerusalem. As I drive around, I spot many other women in the cars around me, who are also struggling to find a parking spot. I can see others making their way on foot from the central bus station, which is just a short walk away. I finally park and join the wave of women walking toward the entrance. Some are walking by themselves, but many have come together in small groups. I take in the colorful dresses, the variety of head coverings—from berets to wigs to big headscarves, which have become more and more visible among the younger generation of Orthodox women. As we approach the entrance and stand in the long line, young girls walk between us to hand out little red bags. I open my little "party bag" and find an array of pamphlets that have been carefully chosen for this crowd—discounts for modest clothing, a small prayer book, and a raffle ticket for Dabri Shir, a Jewish music and book store. I am also equipped with a yellow A4 notebook, accompanied with a pen, signaling that today we have come to learn (and take notes!).

I take a step in and see that the hall has been carefully set up with dozens of round tables adorned with purple flowers. Refreshment stands with cheap coffee and piles of rugelach pastries are spread at numerous locations along the walls. Some young mothers are using this time to breastfeed before they shift the babysitting responsibilities to their older daughters, who have come to watch their young siblings while their mothers attend lectures and workshops. I continue up the stairs and discover an entire hallway filled with stalls of Jewish books, modest clothing, head coverings, and various Judaica.

> Even though Rabbi Ohad Tirosh, one of the organizers of the event, states that "Woman come here to work!," it is very clear that they also have arrived to a quasi festival, where they can meet friends, stock up their wardrobes, and purchase new Jewish-related must-haves, like a new silicone challah-shape pan (designed to help mothers, like me, whose bread-braiding capabilities are minimal). But there is no time for shopping. I continue up the stairs searching for the room where there is a panel about parenting I know I must attend.

This description from my field notes, which I recorded in 2017, offers a depiction of one of the largest annual conferences on "family studies," which was organized by Binyan Shalem, a name that literally means "a complete building." This conference is the main event of the organization, established by Rabbi Ohad and Rabbanit Dana Tirosh in 1998, with the goal to "study family seriously."[8] Though weekly lectures are available throughout the year, the highlight of Binyan Shalem's activities is the yearly summer conference, which is attended by thousands of women, and recently by hundreds of men. Resonating with historian Laura Briggs's attention to how motherhood is cultivated through reproductive labor, these settings foster the notion that women are meant to "work," reinforcing women's pivotal role in making families.[9]

Binyan Shalem is but one of the family-focused education organizations that have been established over the past twenty years along the spectrum of Orthodox communities in Israel. While some focus on premarital preparation, others focus on sexuality and women's health, and still others offer workshops to cultivate better parenting skills. All these events reflect a growing understanding that men and women are ill-prepared for marriage. As we have seen, premarriage classes offer only a basic introduction, so many couples (who have the time and money) further their knowledge through classes and courses, like those offered by Binyan Shalem. These organizations focus on creating alternative settings for Jewish family education, which they view as the only way to safeguard the heterosexual and (re)productive Jewish family, which is under threat, especially from divorce.

While many parenting classes and organizations focused on family well-being and parenting are available in Israel, I have focused my research on individuals, networks, and organizations that self-identify as Jewish in their public presence and attribute at least some of their motivation for assisting parents to their religious ideals. It is also important to note what I mean by Jewish community. First, I tend to use the plural form "communities" when speaking and writing about Orthodox Jews in Israel. There is no such thing as a homogeneous and unified Jewish Orthodox community in Israel (or elsewhere). Even though there is a Jewish rabbinate that is recognized as the supreme rabbinic authority for Judaism in Israel, in practice, the boundaries of these communities are constantly debated. More specifically, in the context of Jewish family education, the driving forces behind these events are individual advocates. Some are linked with established educational institutions; other networks are driven by individual advocates or groups that have come together to educate Jewish couples.

It is not surprising, then, that many institutions compete for followers and funding. Some have succeeded in drawing funding and present themselves as experts in this field, while other individuals and smaller networks come and go, many times because they cannot secure funding or need to reframe their efforts.[10] For example, some educators turn into consultants, offering couples therapy either personally or through a network of therapists, like the Haredi organization Yaner (an acronym for "religious marriage consultants"). Another common avenue is health consultations, especially for women's health, of which the Anglo-Orthodox organization Bishvilayich (literally, "for you") is a typical example, while other organizations merge Jewish law with health and fertility, like the well-known Puah Institute (Puah is the name of a Jewish midwife in Egypt who assisted the births of Jewish children despite Pharaoh's orders).

While some organizations and educators attempt to cater to particular audiences, others aim to offer insights about the Jewish family that go beyond specific religious affiliations and, thus, widen their following. As the director of the Puah Institute told me when we sat in his office: "We are here for everyone!" As he said this, he pointed at all the pictures of rabbis that adorn his office wall—encompassing both Mizrahi and Ashkenazi rabbis affiliated with a spectrum of Orthodox streams (all smiling down at us with divine approval).

In what follows, I offer a critical take on the creative ways educators put forward parenting ideals that are tailored to large families. I show how the particular issues outlined earlier, such as economic struggles, intimacy, and bodily needs, are met with repro-theologies that fuse practical and theological moral governance for managing reproductive lives. As noted previously, by referring to these expressions of Jewish reproductive governance as repro-theologies, I push against the notion that theologies are derived from canonical texts and instead advance a bottom-up understanding of how people come to navigate the gaps between the religious obligation to have a large a family and the extreme difficulties this obligation has come to entail.

## Repro-Theologies of Exhaustion

On a cold Wednesday morning in February 2011, I join the bridal class at a Bais Yaakov seminary in Jerusalem. For an hour, Mrs. Schwartz outlined the practical aspects of homemaking, while giving everyday examples of how to make dinner when you have nothing left in the fridge. Mrs. Schwartz seemed well aware of the difficult realities her students were up against and was offering as much emotional and practical preparation as she could. She began to speak:

> You know, today things are so confusing. You open up *Yated*, and you get so confused.[11] On the one hand, you read the newspaper and see that there is such a need to give [charity]. But then you turn the page and

see all the advertisements for special deals at kosher hotels. And we are confused: should we go on vacation or give charity? This is the confusion we feel as brides and then as mothers. And here I must say something important—your parents got married twenty years ago, and they slowly built their home. What you see now is not the way they started. But, when you get married there is a gap that needs to be overcome. The way to do that is to figure out—what do I really need and what is unnecessary? So, I ask you what is unnecessary?

I watch as the young women offer different answers: a car is unnecessary, as is new furniture, an apartment in Jerusalem, a dryer, a dishwasher, air-conditioning, and a sofa. "But, a sofa is not a luxury!" Rivka objects. Chani responds to her: "At the beginning we can just sit on chairs. A sofa can come later." Mrs. Schwartz smiles proudly and then shares: "I would like to offer a definition our sages have used for luxury. If people were collecting money for it—would you donate your money for the cause? If the answer is no, then it is a luxury."

\* \* \*

During my fieldwork, I participated in many lectures promoting ideologies of simple living. Similarly to Mrs. Schwartz, educators offer practical tips that include time management lessons and work-home balance as well as endless "how-to" guides (e.g., "how to make a beautiful meal when all you have left in the fridge is one tomato"). As part of preparation for married life, educators offer practical tips that are fused with moral guidance on the economic aspects of family life.

In a society where most households struggle with poverty, Mrs. Schwartz offers two practical tools to minimize the gaps between expectations and the economic hardships she knows most of her students are going to face. First, she suggests that her students view the homes they were raised in as products of a long process rather than a starting point. This perspective not only allows them to accept the low economic standards with which they will likely begin their married lives but also shows them a way forward as they make long-term plans to equip their homes slowly, step by step. Second, Mrs. Schwartz opts for a very broad definition of luxury, fusing calculated homemaking with moral discipline. In this way, she offers these young women a start to their journeys with a feeling that they have what they need, and all the other things they may dream of for their home are luxuries that they might succeed in purchasing in the future. Hence, Mrs. Schwartz turns the dire economic situation into an opportunity for frugal living, which serves as a tool to prepare young women for the gaps they will experience between their dreams and their lived realities.

This framework mirrors the belief that successful marriages are a product of individual, and especially female, managerial skills, which are essential to continue to make large families. While most educators steer clear from incorporating economic factors into family planning calculations, their moral governance normalizes the creation of large families who constantly make do with little. These findings mirror the work of Orit Avishai and Jennifer Randles in the United States, which has shown how marriage educators focus on personal and managerial factors instead of addressing the structural and economic foundations of poverty due to failing welfare policies.[12]

Ignoring these neoliberal policy changes was common among Israeli marriage educators, too. Marriage coaches and counselors were more likely to offer psychological tools to assist couples with the constant fights and struggles that are part and parcel of living without enough money to make ends meet. While one-on-one therapy in Israel is relatively costly (250 to 350 shekels per session), many organizations offer cheap group sessions. In these sessions, therapists will frequently pose different challenging case scenarios while suggesting how couples could better react in these types of situations.

Even though marriage counselors tend to focus on the importance of communication skills, their discourse also features moral dilemmas. Yaner, one of the Haredi networks that offers family education and various forms of couple therapy, often addresses these moral topics in its classes and monthly newsletters. For example, in one of the Yaner newsletters, an author poses a question: "Is a father required according to Halacha to pay for healthy food for his children. And, to what extent?" While Jewish law requires parents (predominantly fathers) to provide food for their children, this question reflects how parenting and economic questions are fused with ethical questions that are challenged by modern parenting ideals. The emergence of "healthy" food norms poses not only an economic challenge for large families but also a moral predicament.

Some educators, however, offer a competing strategy to support parents who struggle to manage the gap between what they "should" and what they can offer their children. I found that while educators like Mrs. Schwartz focus on sharpening managerial tools, others actually suggest dropping these tools. One of the most vivid (and humorous) accounts of this approach was shared by Rabbanit Esti, who was invited to give the closing lecture at a full day of learning dedicated to women's health, Jewish law, and technology. Dressed in her usual elegant fashion, wearing a black suit with a black hat adorned with black plastic pearls around the brim, she looked at the hundreds of women in the room and sighed, then spoke:

> I know you are tired. We are all tired. But I must tell you a secret about being tired. According to the Zohar, the most successful children are born from Friday night intimacy.[13] Why? Because then the mother has no strength left. After preparing all the food, preparing the table, cleaning the house . . . she has no strength left. If we look at the Bible, we can see that all the firstborns are the most unsuccessful in the Bible. Why? Because "Kochi vereshit Oni" [My firstborn, my might, the first sign of my strength; Genesis 49:3].
>
> When I had my first child, I said: I will make sure he listens to Baby Mozart music, teach him to read at age two . . . poor kid. Firstborns may be the most successful professionally but they are also an emotional mess, because they are most pressured. The sixth, seventh, eighth child . . . what

kids they turn out to be! They don't get As on their tests, but they have self-confidence and they have many friends. My younger children go to sleep with their backpacks on, searching for a *shidduch* [matchmaker] online.... [Everyone laughs.] You know, I used to take them to the doctor for every cut. Now, my child comes complaining, "Look mother, my hand is falling off," and I say: "It will pass." These children are much healthier and have much more self-confidence. But, controlling motherhood... I tell you, Friday night children... do I still have strength for it? It is great. Exhausted mothers create successful children.

Rabbanit Esti offers a vivid account of what I call a repro-theology of exhaustion. During her lecture, she draws on her own experiences as a mother of nine to convey that she sincerely understands the daily challenges that the women in her crowd are facing. In fact, Rabbanit Esti is a sought-out religious educator, both for her vast knowledge of Jewish texts (which is a rare commodity among Jewish women) and for her ability to interpret texts to mirror and "strengthen" religious women. In this case, through a creative (and humorous) interpretation of Jewish texts, she finds ways to valorize women's reproductive labor. First, while Friday night sex is recommended in Judaism (because it is considered to be part of the Sabbath delight), she shifts the focus from sexual satisfaction to reproduction. By fusing Friday night sex with a zoharic interpretation (which typically offers a mystical reflection on Jewish texts), she also links the time of conception to the personality of the child to be born. In other words, the mother's status of exhaustion is what brings forward "healthy children," as Rabbanit Esti puts it. But she also extends this repro-theology well beyond Friday night as she posits that any "exhausted mother creates successful children." While most of the Jewish texts on motherhood (as rare as they are) typically portray motherhood through male eyes, she is able to reread these texts in ways that resonate with the exhaustion she knows everyone in the room shares.

Rabbanit Esti's interpretation also criticizes "controlling motherhood," referring to contemporary parenting ideals that have been characterized by sociologist Sharon Hays as "intensive motherhood."[14] Rabbanit Esti evokes teaching a child to read prematurely and listening to Baby Mozart (an umbrella term for music and videos that are described as beneficial for toddlers' mental and physical development) as two examples of overambitious parenting. As noted earlier, intensive parenting is hard for large families to adopt, so she frames these practices as examples of unnecessary efforts while promoting "exhausted" Jewish parenting as superior. I argue that this critique offers theological support to mothers who feel that large families do not allow them to fulfill contemporary ideals of intensive motherhood in the context of large families.

As anthropologist Heather Paxson has shown, "motherhood is part of a larger moral economy of gender and kinship in which women are concerned with being 'good' mothers."[15] As Jewish mothers struggle to live up to contemporary parenting models, Jewish educators must put forward new models of how to be a "good" parent in a large family. In a relatable way, Rabbanit Esti draws on her own experience of having children as a process of shedding "controlling ideals," while cultivating a Jewish ethic of "exhausted motherhood" that is viable for large families. Rabbanit Esti, hence, reframes parenting practices that might be deemed neglectful (e.g., disregarding a child who is complaining that his hand is falling off) by repackaging them as positive techniques to cultivate independent children, which she herself models.

In fact, repackaging "neglectful" depictions of large-family practices was common among religious educators and also served as a way to critique shifting state reproductive policies. For example, Mrs. Staestky, a well-known family educator, told a room filled with hundreds of women:

> Once I had the privilege to meet one of the Knesset members. When he found out that I have ten kids he looked at me and said: you and your

family are in charge of the poverty line in Israel. Will you really be able to provide for them? Buy them each an apartment, pay for their college degrees? Not to mention the psychological neglect. So what did I tell him? I told him that he has a very specific attitude as to what parents can give to a child. All you care about is what you can hold in your hand, just like most of the modern world. Do you know how wonderful it is for a child to see that his parents think that he is so wonderful that they want to have another one just like him?

What does a child learn when his parents only have one? That he is a burden. In houses with two children and three computers there are many things missing. What children receive in large families is beyond what they could ever receive in small ones. They learn how to handle different people, how to share. They learn patience and they also learn how to fight. We prepare them to be part of society. They are not going to need to go to psychologists, *your* children are!

At the heart of Mrs. Staestky's critique of modern parenting is a creative reaction to state policy aimed at limiting reproduction in the religious sector and managing demographic growth. As couples struggle to live up to modern parenting ideals (presented by a state they perceive as secular), the creative repro-theologies offered by religious educators aim to reconcile competing reproductive desires in the midst of shifting modes of reproductive governance. In her talk, Mrs. Staestky takes issue with critical "neglect discourses," which are part of the public critiques against high fertility levels among the Orthodox. While these shifting policies were introduced as economic incentives to teach parents that "kids are not work" (as Benjamin Netanyahu put it when he intentionally cut state child support in 2003), this public policy discourse was also fused with critical takes on parental responsibility.

Anthropologists have argued that the work of raising "good" children is a "universal function of the family."[16] As anthropologist Cheryl Mattingly put it, the family can also be a courtroom, where parents are "judged" for their successes and their failures.[17] The history of reproduction in Israel, as noted earlier, is paved with racialized and anti-religious sentiments toward the high fertility rates of religious and racialized Mizrahi Jews. By offering this carefully crafted answer to a member of the Israeli Knesset, Mrs. Staestky is providing tools to combat this discourse. In turn, these creative interpretations resist the stigma of neglect in large families.

But she knows, as do all the other women in the room, that this struggle is not merely an external dispute. She is also offering the women tools to resist their emerging desires, making sure these external critiques are not taken too much to heart. As couples debate whether (and how) to continue their desires to have large families, Mrs. Staestky offers tools to combat the critical voices from within that are "dangerously" eating away at these ideals.

## Intimacy versus Reproduction

One of the other "dangers" educators often combat is the cost of large-family life on intimacy. Early marriages that are predominantly focused on reproduction do not allow couples to "just be a couple," as Moshe put it. In the Haredi context, where couples date for only a short amount of time—typically a few months with little if any physical closeness before marriage—intimacy only comes with time and effort, which is not easily available. While Religious Zionist couples often date longer, which sometimes involves partial sexual intimacy, educators tend to gravitate toward belittling the importance of couple intimacy as a goal in itself. As anthropologist Ari Engelberg has shown, even though Religious Zionist dating norms encourage ideals of romantic love, many rabbis and educators "adopt the Ultra-Orthodox ideology that views romantic love as superfluous."[18]

In an attempt to assist couples to form meaningful relationships, Haredi educators, and especially couple therapists, offer various tools. As Moshe, one of the consultants, explained at one of the lectures I observed:

> When we get married, we must change the ways we think. We are used to being individuals that typically listen to our parents. When we get married we need to learn that we are together. In our clinic we see couples who really struggle with creating intimacy. The men are used to having *chavrutot* [study partners]. That is what they know about friendship. And, until now, they have chosen their friends based on—who can help me get smarter? Who can make my mind sharper? Who can I have philosophical conversations with? And, with this experience, you get married. And your wife tells you to do one, two, three . . . and you answer her: But who said? Who said you need to put three eggs in? I am telling you that this is what kills your relationship!

Moshe, an experienced Haredi couple therapist, considers gendered separation norms to be the source of a rocky start for married life. In a society where friendships are cultivated only among members of the same sex, married life is the first time men and women seek to cultivate real friendships. More specifically, Moshe points to a gap between male friendship, which is crafted around Torah study,[19] and couple intimacy, which requires a different framework. Whereas Torah study is characterized by constant questioning and philosophical debates, sharing household-related tasks does not require philosophical deliberations. According to Moshe, it is this "gap" that creates communication difficulty that "kills" relationships.

Whereas Moshe attempts to manage the desire for intimacy by offering communication skills, other educators criticize the overemphasis on intimacy as the trouble in itself. As Rabbanit Miriam described:

> In the Torah, intimacy is a side effect of children. The important thing is the pregnancy . . . in the Bible, intimacy is not a supreme principle. Are men a side effect? [She nods her head and all the women laugh.] In our generation, intimacy has become the highest value. We have lost our honor because we have turned intimacy into our idols. . . . The Rav Kook said it beautifully. Rachel died early because intimacy was the most im-

portant to her and that's why she died during childbirth. Whereas, Leah had unlimited eyesight, she looks ahead and that is why the Messiah will come from her.

Rabbanit Miriam offers a creative interpretation of attitudes toward fertility among two Jewish matriarchs, who both struggle with different aspects of reproduction.[20] Based on the writings of Rabbi Abraham Isaac Kook, one the founders of Religious Zionism, she creates two ideal types comparing Rachel, who yearns for intimacy, to Leah, who focuses on child-rearing and bears six children to Jacob. Offering a critical cause for Rachel's death, she explains that Rachel's decision to pursue intimacy cost her her life, which metaphorically plays out by her death during the birth of her second son. Rabbanit Miriam uses this binary model to criticize contemporary ideas that overemphasize the importance of intimacy as idol worship. In this framework, fertility and family life are put in the center, sometimes even at the expense of putting men (and intimacy) out of the picture. In doing so, Rabbanit Miriam's repro-theology offers a creative strategy to keep the desire for a large family intact by reverting the desire for intimacy back to the one and only important desire: to have children.

## Healthy Hungers

In light of the various hardships they face, many couples wonder whether it would have been better to wait and build intimacy and more financial stability before having children. In response to this growing issue, educators have been pushed to offer new rationalizations to explicitly promote and support early marriage, regardless of the challenges discussed earlier. First and foremost, educators stress that young marriage is the best path to enable healthy pregnancies, which are the prerequisite for large families. Dr. Chana Katan, the well-known religious gynecologist mentioned earlier, and her husband, Rabbi Yoel Katan, are prominent figures in the national-religious Zionist stream who are both public promoters of this ideology. As a couple who combine both medical and rabbinic "spheres of authority,"[21] they frequently lecture and write, both together and separately, to promote early marriages. According to them, not only is early marriage a religious ideal, but "the biological clock ticks according to halacha," they often say while fusing Jewish law and biology. Statistical information is also utilized to ground the reality in which having children early is the best possible method to bear large families as fertility declines with age. In light of the growth of global infertility,[22] repro-theology mobilizes statistics as its promoters claim that the best way to counter infertility is to marry early and to immediately have as many children as possible.

Yet, promoting early marriage and reproduction usually means that married couples start their family life at the same time that they begin their professional training. This issue is twofold as it affects both the household income and the stress on the young parents, especially the mother, who needs to focus simultaneously on child-rearing and building a career, a common predicament scholars have documented all over the world.[23] In the Jewish context, this pronatal ideal continues to create significant constraints on the female body and the couple's everyday life, as well as contributing to the financial difficulties described earlier. Constructing a contemporary repro-theology that takes these struggles into account, many educators describe building a family as a mission or as a challenge.[24] They often compare the "family-building" challenge to other temptations of the evil inclination, which both acknowledges the gravity of the struggles couples face and turns these "quests for conception" into sacred quests.[25] In her guide to newlyweds, Dr. Chana Katan acknowledges these hardships by offering creative and practical ideas to assist young couples:

> We must remember that some of these dear women live in far settlements, many of them travel several hours to study, often hitchhiking rides to get there. These conditions, adding to regular house chores, create deep fatigue. Many times these young women do not find time (and strength) to make healthy food and to attend their periodical medical visits. It is at

this point that the husband (who is also just a young bird) should accept upon himself to supervise over the nutrition of his young wife and make sure she balances between her many tasks in favor of her health and the health of the future child. Sometimes it is good to recruit a third responsible person to "adopt" the couple—a parent, an older brother, a rabbi, or a doctor—to keep an eye out for them.[26]

In her description, Dr. Katan clearly acknowledges the challenges these conditions create. To counter them, she suggests additional supervision over the woman's health through either the husband or other paternalistic figures, such as a parent, older brother, rabbi, or doctor. The "dear woman" is portrayed as a person who cannot make the healthy decisions that are needed, and she is therefore assigned to the supervision of patrons to make sure she reaches the finish line as a healthy mother to a healthy baby.

This heightened governance of the reproductive body came up constantly in the talks I attended. A vivid example was offered at one of the conferences I joined where a dietitian named Michal was invited to discuss the topic "How to Prepare for a Pregnancy." At the beginning of her presentation, she states, "We must remember that when we are pregnant we are going to war," and then asks the room filled with women, "Who are we fighting?" One woman calls out, "Hormones," and everyone laughs. To this, Michal answers:

We are fighting everything that is pulling us down—nausea, tiredness, sweet inclinations. . . . We must fight back and not give in. One of the secrets of success for a pregnancy is to plan them. But, you know, we don't usually plan our pregnancies (everyone laughs). It might be more precise to say that we never plan our pregnancies, which is why they are always at such a bad time . . . but once we know we are pregnant we must prepare. During our fertile years, we must always eat well and make sure to lead a healthy life. What I always say is: "Depart from evil and do good." Even if we don't succeed to stay away from sugar and coffee, we can always do

> the good—eat more fruit and vegetables. The Ministry of Health recommends to eat five to eight fruits a day. Yes! Not the ministry of veganism—the Ministry of Health. If you could even do that, you would feel much better. You can make a shake every day. I am telling you—eat well and you won't feel nausea. Our body doesn't really need help, it knows what to do, we just need to give it strength.

As part of a two-hour lecture on healthy eating to support healthy pregnancies, Michal offers detailed examples of foods that can help pregnancies go along better. She acknowledges the difficulties women encounter during their pregnancies and utilizes a vocabulary of battle to combat these difficulties. As noted earlier, in contrast to the vast literature on nationalist discourses of reproduction in Israel,[27] I found that educators rarely inspired Orthodox couples through post-Holocaust and Zionist ideals. Michal's narrative is a vivid example of the other "wars" women are facing. Michal, like many of the other educators I met, inspired couples to stay on the large-family track by focusing on practical remedies to solve existential and everyday difficulties. To put it simply, there is no need to plan your pregnancies, a stance reflecting the common anti-family planning discourse. What is crucial, however, is to make a meal plan. To substantiate her claim, Michal refers to Psalms 34:14, "Depart from evil and do good," a quotation that is often referred to in moral aspects of Jewish praxis. The contours of this praxis are constructed vis-à-vis growing veganism trends in Israel, which are often conflated with "secular" ideologies. Resonating with Marie Griffith's work in the Evangelical context where women decide to "become slim for him,"[28] linking morality to the management of the pregnant body instills this "war" with religiosity. According to this repro-theology, pregnancies are always a given, yet the reproductive labor is linked to how much you prepare your body for it.

## Family Planning as a Holy Obligation?

While many of the educators offered creative and often paternalistic projects for governing the reproductive body, there were also educators who created spaces to critique the large-family ideals. One morning, I joined Rabbanit Kahn, one of the most vocal critics of the large-family ideology, at a lecture she gave to a women's learning group in southern Israel. Rabbanit Kahn handed out papers that listed Jewish sources on reproduction for each group to learn together with *chavrutot* (study partners), and then she offered the following comments:

> After you have learned the sources about family planning, I think the question we must ask is, why does the Talmud bring the story of Rabbi Chiya's wife to prove that women are exempt from the obligation to "be fertile and reproduce"?[29] I think that it shows us that the exemption of women from this obligation was based on one woman who found childbearing unbearable. You know, many women are bothered by this exemption of women, I say that it is the exact opposite—it shows us how wise our sages are! Our sages learn from this story that women do not have an obligation to have children, maybe a small obligation to try and help their husbands. That is it.

At this point, a woman in the room calls out, "But this can't be! People consult with rabbis and you hear that rabbis tell women to have children even when they already have six children or when people are sick, even when they have cancer!"

This encounter reflects an intriguing phenomenon. Rabbanit Kahn comes to learn the canonical texts on family planning with a group of women. This type of *chavruta*-style Talmud study for women is a rather common phenomenon in modern-Orthodox settings, but it is still at the margins of ultra-Orthodoxy. Rabbanit Kahn offers an interpretation of the texts that exempts women from procreation, an interpretation that is in accordance with mainstream Jewish law (even though it has been the subject of feminist critique for decades).³⁰ However, the women in her class are surprised by this interpretation because it runs contrary to the accepted norms in their communities to have large families at any cost. Rabbanit Kahn addresses this dissonance as follows:

> I am about to say some radical things. You know, rabbis who don't tell women that they are exempt from procreation and maybe only obligated to help their husbands are committing the four following sins: "Love your neighbor," "A person shall not afflict his fellow," "You shall not stand idly by the shedding of the blood of thy fellow," and maybe even "Before the blind"! Do you understand this? In order to promote one *mitzvah derabanan* [of our rabbis] they go against four obligations of *deorayta* [of the written Torah]!

During her lecture, Rabbanit Kahn deeply critiques contemporary pronatal norms that are reinforced by rigid rabbinic guidelines. She creatively uses a Jewish legal framework to criticize rabbis who do not tell women that they are exempt from procreation with a handful of sins. In Jewish law, a law is considered *deorayta* (Aramaic: דאורייתא, "of the Torah,") if it was given with the written Torah. In contrast, a law is considered *derabanan* (Aramaic: דרבנן, "of our rabbis," or rabbinic) if it is ordained by the rabbinic sages. It is often unclear whether a religious obligation is *deorayta* or *derabanan*—these terms are used extensively in Jewish law, where lengthy debates often surface. These legal distinctions have extensive ramifications in terms of religious observance, the severity of sin, and so forth. In Rabbanit Kahn's framing, she posits one religious obligation that is considered to be *deorayta* (of the Torah), in contrast to three other obligations that are typically considered to be *derabanan* (rabbinic). Her interpretative work uses traditional Jewish law categories to challenge the legal status of the obligation to have many children at all costs.

This critical and studious discourse surfaced in some of the classes I attended, primarily those taught by female (especially among Religious

Zionist) educators in less institutionalized settings. In 2014, Rabbanit Malka Puterkovsky published a book that carefully describes this ideology, generating a public discussion of what had until then been a private and hushed discourse.[31] In her book, Puterkovsky frames parenthood as a hard and satisfying mission that men, and especially women, take upon themselves. However, she describes the ramifications of this mission on couples who pursue this undertaking without knowing that family planning is a viable option. Child after child, emotional and economic stress grows, often translating into marital trouble, which has led Puterkovsky to transform her opinion regarding family planning: "Today, my opinion is that family planning is a holy obligation, no less. . . . I am not willing to be satisfied with any less than a deep yearning to bring a child to the world."[32]

This ideological transformation has led Rabbanit Puterkovsky to become an active and vocal critic of the common discourse "we never plan children," described earlier. In return, Puterkovsky was publicly critiqued by some of the public figures described in this book, including Dr. Chana and Rabbi Yoel Katan.[33] According to Rabbanit Puterkovsky, children should not be conceived mindlessly, but as a product of deep yearning. Religious obligation was portrayed as the main motivation for having children, but Puterkovsky focused on desire as the sole reason to have children. While other educators propose organization and emotional management of pregnancies, Puterkovsky writes that it is only a deep desire that can assist couples in overcoming the real challenges of building a family:

> In our generation, the challenges of family building are more complicated, in my opinion, than ever before. This has many reasons, I will mention only a few here: changes in the status of women, women's motivation to use their strengths and offer their unique strengths to the whole world (also outside of the house), the economic need for income from both spouses. . . . Also, couples who want to bring up their children with devotion and faith must spend a lot of time and strength focusing on

their education in light of the processes that characterize our generation: the loss of parental authority, consumption of "dirty culture," physical, psychological, and sexual abuse of children, the addiction to computer screens and other technological machines.[34]

The challenges of parenthood today, Rabbanit Puterkovsky argues, must be met with a reorientation of reproductive norms. To solidify her position, she offers a creative reading of the canonical sources on reproduction, while specifically focusing on the exemption of women from the obligation to "be fruitful and multiply." Her position works on two premises. First, she shows that women are exempt from procreation and may use birth control for any reason they desire. As she puts it elsewhere: "In such a complicated and sensitive subject like pregnancy and childbirth can one ignore the fact that women should decide when to help their husbands with his obligation?"[35] Second, she addresses the husband's obligation to have children by embracing the term *shihuy mitzvah* (literally, "to postpone a mitzvah"),[36] arguing that postponing a mitzvah to perform it better in the future is preferable. In other words, the quantity of children is not the only end game:

> Who may decide what a body can or can't handle? Is there an objective scale for a Jewish scholar to decide? . . . The suffering caused by becoming parents before feeling secure in marriage is included in the halachic category of "A person shall not afflict his fellow." Furthermore, an unwanted child goes against the basic principle "Love your neighbor." Even the strictest Jewish legal scholar would not wish to be born unwanted.[37]

Crafting together well-known principles such as "A person shall not afflict his fellow" and "Love your neighbor as yourself," she intentionally links them to family planning. These creative ideas show the extent to which she goes to find support in Jewish law for her position. It also reflects her deep criticism of the power Jewish authorities have taken on these issues, a critique Michal Raucher has well documented in her work.³⁸ Amid prevalent norms in which having children is a "natural" outcome, she pushes for a renewed orientation of reproductive desire. It is not that she does not want people to have children; instead, Rabbanit Puterkovsky begs people to truly desire to have them.

\* \* \*

Repro-theologies can be used to either challenge or reinforce having large families. Couples encounter these competing narratives as they consider their reproductive futures amid growing economic, social, and bodily difficulties. Repro-theologies are not limited to canonical Jewish texts. They are shaped by various mediators of Jewish knowledge who fuse practical, emotional, and theological notions with creative interpretations of Jewish texts as they try to help couples combat emerging desires that threaten the large-family telos or as they assist couples to reorient their desires toward new horizons.

Educators who espouse repro-theologies offer creative, and often critical, ways to address some of the cracks that shape family-making decisions in Orthodox communities: the economic difficulties linked to early marriages and the tolls these take on couple intimacy, work-family balance, and the female body. While some of these educators use these repro-theologies to push couples to continue on normative lines of pro-natal desires, others, like Rabbanit Malka Puterkovsky, seek to cultivate new forms of parental desire that take personal capabilities and structural challenges into account.

What is not addressed in these educational settings is also notable. As mentioned previously, in contrast to the vast literature on the politics of reproduction in Israel, I found that educators rarely drew upon post-Holocaust or Zionist ideals in their strategies to support Orthodox couples; it was far more common for educators to draw upon existential and everyday difficulties familiar to these communities. In fact, due to robust scholarship on the centrality of nationalist ideologies in reproductive politics, I began to wonder if I was missing something, so I decided to ask some of my interviewees. I was surprised at the following answer I received: "Do you think that is a good reason to have a child? Having a child to win a war with the Arabs? What a terrible thought!" Whereas nationalism seemed to be a powerful source of motivation in the reproductive politics elemental to establishing the Israeli state, this does not seem to be the case among contemporary repro-theologies in Orthodox communities.[39] Contemporary educators put forward more individualistic sources of inspiration that offer creative ways to combat the real "wars" couples are currently fighting.

Still, for many of the couples with whom I spoke, these classes were not enough. Sometimes couples, and especially women, would find support and solace, as well as practical tools that helped them become the better parents and spouses they wanted to be. A very charismatic and uplifting class might equip a mother with a burst of energy for a few days, but eventually the question that the young mother asked at the beginning of this chapter would resurface: "How do I find the strength to continue?" This chapter clearly demonstrates how many of these educational settings are inhabited by very passionate educators whose primary aim is to strengthen the desire (and sharpen one's tools) to succeed in having large families. But what about the women who realize that "more work" might not solve their conflicting desires? These findings also showcase how these spaces primarily speak to a female crowd. But what about the men who are also struggling in the face of harsh realities? The next chapter charts how rabbinic consultation is the perfect place for both men and women.

3

# Creating an Ethical Language

I visited Rachel, a Bais Yaakov seminary teacher, at her home on the outskirts of Jerusalem in 2015. As she chops vegetables in her kitchen, she shares how her dreams were fulfilled when she married a Torah scholar. "It all happened so quickly, I got pregnant immediately. Child after child. Boy after boy. Finally, I had a girl. I was so happy. Now I have someone to help me," she says, smiling. We move on with the story. She stops, then says, "I am debating if I should have another one." She is forty-one and has eleven children, so I was sure she was done. But she elaborates further: "It is so hard. I have been teaching at the seminary and also offering individual classes to other women. I struggle to maintain a household, care for the kids, and also teach. I am not sure—who am I supposed to contribute to? My family or my students? I am not sure. I think I will go and see my rabbi soon." "Soon?" I ask her. "I need him to decide for me," she explains. She grins at me and adds, "But I will decide when to ask him. You see, I have to be ready to accept his opinion."

Unsure whether she should have another child, Rachel plans to seek rabbinic consultation to assist in her reproductive decision-making. Similar to many of the other couples with whom I spoke, she pursues rabbinic authorities to make her decisions, but she does so at her own pace and on her own terms. Throughout this research, I repeatedly met people who told me stories about their encounters with rabbinic figures that did not seem to fit the literature I was familiar with on religious authority. Since Max Weber's classic typology of religious authority, the other models that followed were mostly about submission, and these models did not seem to fit with the (almost) playful attitude Rachel displayed.

Religious authority has been challenged in recent years by members of faith groups due to increasing levels of access to canonical texts through digital media, growing demands for gender justice and pushback against religious patriarchy, and transnational migration patterns, which trouble local notions of religious authority. Anthropologists have noted the ways religious authorities and institutions construct novel models of authoritative knowledge, legitimacy, and power in the face of these mounting contestations.[1] Ayala Fader's work on Hasidic Jews in Brooklyn offers a vivid example of the innovative ways religious authority is legitimated and performed by communal leaders in their public faith talks.[2] She describes how Hasidic rabbis delineate separate "spheres of authority" as they constitute their religious authority vis-à-vis the medical authority of mental health professionals.[3] In the Muslim context, Morgan Clarke demonstrates how Lebanon's Islamic legal experts use digital communication technologies to "facilitate the continuing mobilization of personalized religious authority within and between modern bureaucratic-legal nation-states."[4]

While these studies demonstrate the powerful strategies used to legitimize religious leadership, few studies have highlighted the variety of ways individuals engage with religious authorities in their everyday lives. Houssain Ali Agrama argues that this literature gap is a product of an "imagined binary opposition" between religious authority and ethical agency in "Western" and neoliberal thought.[5] The idea that a true self must be a free self and that freedom consists of following aspirations that originate (solely) in one's self is perceived to automatically turn any mode of willing obedience into a paradox. Following this mode of thought, all types of religious authority appear paradoxical and antithetical to "true" freedom. Accordingly, tradition or authority has been largely perceived as an obstacle to ethical self-formation as "a disposition toward or susceptibility to authority is necessarily antithetical to true agency."[6] In contrast to this approach, Agrama focuses on the shared responsibility that emerges between the fatwa seeker and the mufti to problematize the "liberal" dichotomy between religious authority and ethical agency. Building on Foucauldian frameworks of self-making,[7] Agrama posits that ethical freedom should be perceived as not only in opposition to authority "but rather an expression of it."[8]

As part of this ethical turn in anthropology, the analysis in this chapter builds on Hussain Ali Agrama's work on fatwa-seeking as a shared project of ethical self-making. In what follows, I examine the variety of ways in which Orthodox Jews engage with rabbinic authorities as part of their reproductive decision-making. While the decision to seek personal rabbinic consultation is not a surprising one, it is not obligatory. Even though Jewish law includes rulings on almost every imaginable realm, there has been an ongoing debate about the role rabbis should, could, or are required to take in various dimensions of life. As I analyzed my findings, I was surprised by the prominent role rabbinic consultation still plays in contraception, particularly because religious authority has been seriously challenged in Israeli Orthodoxy in recent years.

The challenges to religious authority have come from a variety of fronts. First, some well-established and widely accepted Jewish scholars have passed away during the past few years, leaving disputes over future leaders and a fragmented structure of rabbinic authority.[9] Thus, men and women may turn for advice to a local community rabbi or a yeshiva-based Torah scholar, or seek advice from a particular rabbi with expertise in a specific area of Jewish law. Second, due to a considerable growth in yeshiva study in Israel, many men have reached high levels of literacy,[10] thus lessening the need to seek advice from others. Also, internet forums enable religious members to address their questions to a large array of rabbinic scholars.[11] These technological advancements, together with a blur in communal borders, trouble local notions of religious authority,[12] and the possibility of moving among communities, customs, norms, and rabbinic styles has greatly increased.

Critiques of rabbinic authority are also emerging as women rethink and challenge the traditional link between male rabbis and religious rulings, especially regarding women's autonomy around reproductive deci-

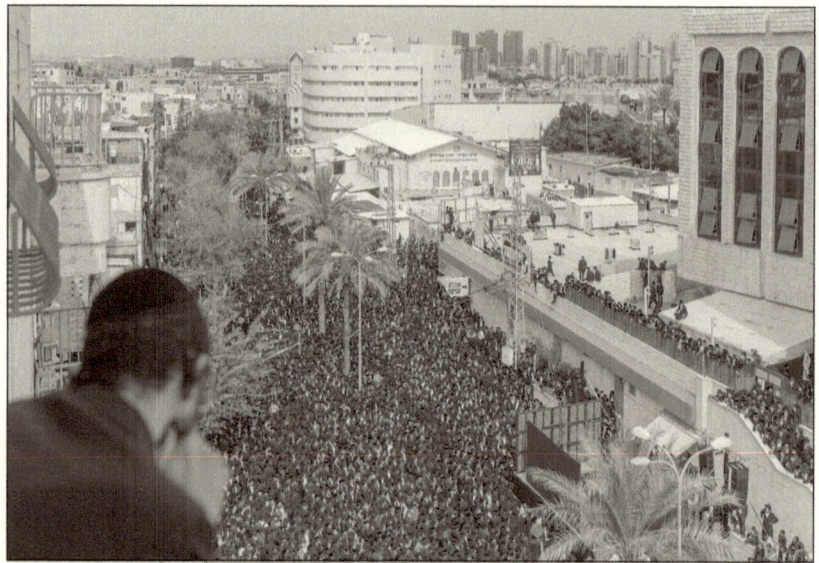

FIGURE 3.1. Hundreds of thousands attend the funeral of Rabbi Chaim Kanievsky, Bnei Brak, Israel, March 20, 2022. Photo by Avishag Shaar-Yashuv.

sions.[13] As the phenomenon of female scholars grows together with a substantial scholarship of feminist critiques of rabbinic legal discourse,[14] vocal calls to "get rabbis out of our womb" are slowly growing. In my own work, I have demonstrated the gendered aspects of authoritative knowledge across the continuum of Jewish Orthodoxy, highlighting how women are interpreting and reinterpreting religious texts to articulate rights to sexual and reproductive autonomy in ways that engender new frameworks of religious authority.[15]

Amid these challenges to rabbinic authority, I wondered why couples were still attracted to the idea of bringing their contraception debates to rabbis. This question only deepened as I found that they did not even always listen to the rabbis they consulted. I determined that Orthodox couples use Jewish law as an ethical compass of reorientation in the midst of moral conflict. Further, I found that for many of my interlocutors, the process of consultation was more significant than rote submission to religious rulings. As we will see, some couples "shop around" until they find a ruling that is to their liking. Some seek to fully accept and submit to religious rulings, while delegating their weighty decisions to rabbis. Others seek the authority of religious figures, yet negotiate the outcomes, either embracing or rejecting rulings while taking their own preferences into account.

Departing from classic debates regarding how religious leaders struggle to legitimate their authority in the eyes of their communities, I turn the lens of anthropological inquiry to the ways in which religious members engage with authorities in their everyday lives. I argue that the analysis of engagement with religious authorities requires attention to inner diversity and the wide range of interpretations and practices within Orthodoxy. Without such attention, anthropologists have propagated an overly harmonious, ideological, and flattened picture of religious consultation. I also flag the importance of temporality, suggesting that religious consultation is reworked over the life course. While religious consultation may offer an ethical language and compass, especially for couples at the beginning stages of marriage, religious authority can also be unlearned as life experiences challenge the relevance of rabbinic rulings.

## Rabbinic Consultation as an Ethical Compass

I first realized how important religious consultation can be when I spoke to Sarah and Moshe. Sarah is a hardworking nurse who was thirty-eight when we spoke; her husband, Moshe, who is one year older, is a schoolteacher. They married in their early twenties and live with their seven children in the growing Haredi settlement of Betar Illit, roughly ten kilometers south of Jerusalem. They moved there right after they got married in order to afford married life but stay close to their parents, who all live in (very expensive) Jerusalem. As they shared their reproductive story with me, they recalled how they decided to consult with a rabbi after the birth of their fourth child. As Sarah put it:

After four children in four and a half years, I felt that I was going to fall apart. Physically, I had no strength left. We went to the rabbi and he told me to go and ask a doctor. Whatever the doctor says—that will be my *pesak* [Jewish law]. I went to the doctor, and do you know what he told me? He said: "Four children in four and a half years? Can you imagine what your body has gone through? You must wait three years until your next child!"

"Must?" I asked. "Must!" I went home very happy that day. But, you know what, after half a year I felt a deep urge to have another child. So, I got pregnant. A few weeks later, I had a miscarriage. It was from heaven. I understood that when the doctor told me three years it really was a *pesak*. And I had not listened. So, I waited, and three years later I had a baby. A healthy baby to a healthy mother.

What struck me about Sarah's account is how hard she works to constantly reinterpret the rabbinic ruling she was given. After four consecutive births, the couple turns to a rabbi who, in turn, sends them to see a physician. Building on Fader's notion of "spheres of authority,"[16] a referral to a medical professional could be perceived as a division of labor between rabbinic and medical authority.[17] Yet, Sarah does not wish to make a distinction between these two forms of authority. On the contrary, she creatively reinterprets the ruling to mean that the rabbi had turned the medical consultation into a sacred, heavenly, and binding authority. Thus, Sarah interprets her miscarriage as a consequence of not listening to her rabbi. By reinterpreting the rabbinic ruling in this way, she makes a concerted effort to ensure that rabbinic rulings remain relevant even as life events challenge the rulings offered. It is through this embodied experience of loss that she reinterprets the meaning of the original ruling, which redefines and strengthens her rabbinic adherence and her obedience to medical authority.

Not all couples I met were so enthusiastic about the relevance of rabbinic rulings to their struggles. In stark contrast to Sarah and Moshe, Chava (forty-two) and Avraham (forty-four), a Dati (Religious Zionist) couple with seven children, also went to talk to a rabbi after the birth of their third child, but they left the meeting disappointed. As Chava described:

> After we had three boys quickly, we went to ask to have a break because we hadn't fulfilled the obligation to "be fruitful," as we didn't have a girl yet. The answers we got were, let's say . . . not satisfactory. Meaning, we didn't get permission. This was hard for us. . . . We discussed this for a while and . . . well, decided to make a judgment ourselves. There was a limit to our strength. We looked into it ourselves, searched online, and realized that after you have one child, you have already completed most of the obligation, which also makes planning a bit easier.

According to Jewish law, it is ideal to have a boy and a girl in order to fulfill the religious obligation "to be fruitful." After having three boys, Chava and Avraham were struggling to take care of their young children and so they looked for permission to take a break. Having received a negative answer, they were put in a difficult position. On the one hand, they had already asked for a rabbinic opinion; on the other, they realized they did not have the strength to have another child. Even though their narrative reflects submissive prenotions of rabbinic authority, an online search broadened the horizon of their possibilities, and they decided to disregard the ruling that they had already been given. In other words, Chava and Avraham negotiated the authority of religious rulings and rejected it when they perceived following it to be unattainable.

Some couples, however, had less "binding" notions of rabbinic rulings from the start. I met Libby, a thirty-one-year-old kindergarten teacher, and Herschel, a thirty-three-year-old Haredi (ultra-Orthodox) yeshiva student at their home in Jerusalem on a warm day in the middle of June. As their children played in the corridor of their tiny apartment, Libby described how after the birth of their first child they were "unsure if they should wait a bit." Libby shared how she read some marriage guidebooks and even attended one class, but they were still unsure. Herschel continued with a smile: "I thought this was a great opportunity to speak to some of the rabbis at my yeshiva, as well as our communal rabbi. So, I set up meetings and went to talk to each and every one of them. It was great. We had good conversations together until I found the opinion that worked best for me." Herschel's playful description of rabbinic consultation offers a vivid depiction of "rabbi shopping," a term I use to describe a common practice to "shop" for the most preferable rabbinic opinion. As I encountered this phenomenon over and over, I wondered: What is the purpose of this type of consultation?

I found that this type of engagement with religious authorities was motivated by a need to create an ethical environment in which to converse. In a community where sexuality is addressed in hushed tones, the determination of reproduction and contraception as a realm of religious consultation creates a "kosher" place to begin to speak. Medical anthropologist Tsipy Ivry has described how medical procedures regarding assisted reproduction are designated "kosher" through a dual process of medicalization of Jewish law, on the one hand, and making medical knowledge "kosher," on the other.[18] While "kosher" is a concept primarily used to designate the kinds of foods Jews are permitted to eat, medical procedures are designated "kosher" through rabbinic biomedical knowledge. Building on these insights, I argue that ethical or "kosher" decisions are not rendered solely by their outcomes but by the particular contexts through which decisions emerge. It is through the process of sharing decisions with rabbis that taboo-like conversations become "kosher."

Rabbinic consultation also allows for a language to speak about silenced taboos. During my fieldwork, the word "contraception" rarely surfaced. Contraception was constantly referred to as *zeh* (Hebrew for "it"), or merely as "prevention," or "planning" without any specification. As couples search for ways to discuss "it," consulting with a rabbi entails the use of a Jewish legal framework, which in itself offers a language. While halacha (Jewish law) is typically described as a system of law, for the couples I met, it provided an ethical language.

But there were couples who sought more than an ethical language. On a cold Wednesday evening, I met Naomi and Elad, a Dati couple, at their home in northern Israel. Elad (thirty-eight), an engineer, and Naomi (thirty-five), a physical therapist, were expecting their third child at the time of our meeting. As we sat on their porch, I watched Naomi's smile as she placed her hands on her stomach, but I could tell there was something that was making them uncomfortable as they recalled their initial steps into parenthood. Finally, Elad broke the silence:

> We went to India after our wedding for a few months, and Naomi came back pregnant. We didn't think it was a big deal that we had waited a few months, but then we went to the doctor . . . there was something wrong with the baby. We went from ultrasound to ultrasound. They didn't think she would live to reach her first birthday. We were shocked. We didn't know what to do.

Naomi continued the story:

> We spent the next month going to different specialists but also looking for spiritual guidance. We prayed so much. And went to different rabbis. Some said we should just have faith and that doctors make mistakes all the time . . . but there was one rabbi, a rabbi who specialized in medicine, and he changed everything for us. He asked us to bring all the materials with us, and we sat together for a long time. At the end, he looked at us and said, "I am not giving you a choice. You need to abort this baby."

Elad said, "I remembered I was shocked by this. How could he make such a decision? But, you know what? I was somehow comforted by it." Naomi agreed. "It was exactly what I needed to hear. I needed someone with broad shoulders to take the weight off my shoulders."

Naomi and Elad's tragedy came to me as a surprise. As I listened to the story of their journey to parenthood, I was struck by the central role rabbinic consultation played in their decision-making process, especially as they were critical about various aspects of religious life throughout the interview, reflecting a flexible orthopraxis that selectively followed religious strictures. Further, their narrative reflects a paradoxical situation: on the one hand, they shop around until they get an answer they can accept. On the other, once they find the opinion they are comfortable with, they are ready to fully submit to this ruling. The emic term "broad shoulders," which is widely used to describe esteemed rabbinic scholars, hinting at a hierarchy of expertise, reflects how they wish to defer their personal responsibility to a rabbinic expert. At this moment in their life, the rabbi with "broad shoulders," who demands to take the burden off their shoulders, was "exactly what they needed." This moral division of labor also reflects an important tendency to share decision-making with authoritative others, especially amid tough decisions.[19]

### Rabbis as (Powerful) Mediators

Despite the harmonious front that appears in many of the narratives I have shared in this book, I often found that couples were at odds with each other. Debates about their shared trajectory of family life were sprinkled with big ethical, emotional, theological, and technical questions, and they did not always agree regarding the steps they should take. Even though they were both struggling, sometimes the women were the ones who wanted to continue to have more children while their husbands were convinced it was best to take a break, and sometimes the opposite was true.

Amid these debates, I found that religious consultation also serves as a space of authoritative mediation for debating couples. Ayelet and Shimmy's story illustrates this complex situation. I met Ayelet and Shimmy at their house on a Friday afternoon. Shimmy (thirty-two), an education consultant at a local school, and Ayelet (twenty-nine), a self-employed graphic designer, reside in a Religious Zionist settlement in the West Bank. After their engagement, they sought rabbinic consultation, as Shimmy wanted children immediately, but Ayelet was rather young and unsure. Shimmy and Ayelet took their debate to Shimmy's rabbi as a way of inviting an authoritative mediator into their personal conflict.

> AYELET: "We went to speak with Rav Meron. And . . . he said no to waiting. First, he listened to us. He wanted to hear why. Then he explained why he thinks a couple should have a first child and wait after we have a first child. He spoke about it as being a gift.
> SHIMMY: I would tell the same story with a different tune. It did not start with a "no." It started from him listening. He wanted to understand why. What our debates were. I don't remember it as a binding *pesak*. I don't remember him saying we weren't allowed. I remember him saying, "This is what I think. And you decide."
> AYELET: I got into this marriage quickly. I am happy I never had years of endless searching. But I wanted to stabilize the marriage for a few months before having children. When we went to the rabbi, I felt that the way he talked about it meant that there was not really any other option. This is what you are supposed to do. And that is what we did. So we got married and I was pregnant a month later. It was really hard. I was in total shock. I was sure my life was over. I sat and cried for days. It was terrible. I just got married. I have no idea what I want to do with my life. And I am about to be a mother. Shimmy didn't know what to do with me.
> SHIMMY: I remember being very surprised by your reaction. I was in the kitchen in the caravan. You told me and sat down and started crying. I really remember that. I was so surprised. We debated about it, we spoke to Rav Meron and we had made a decision . . .
> AYELET: Yes. *We* made a decision.

While analyzing Ayelet and Shimmy's story, I quickly realized that consultation with a rabbinic authority was an encounter they experienced differently. Even though "no" is quite a definitive (and powerful) word, the meaning of this rabbinic ruling was understood differently by Ayelet and Shimmy. Ayelet perceived this encounter as a *pesak*—that is, a binding ruling of Jewish law—while Shimmy regarded it more like an opinion. Nevertheless, they made a choice based on this (different) encounter. Or rather, Shimmy made a choice. Ayelet is sarcastic about this decision that she had only partially made.

Yet, this was not merely a personal variance. These encounters reflected and permeated a particular gendered configuration of authoritative knowledge. This structural asymmetry was a result of factors that create different systems and access to religious knowledge for men and women within the Jewish Orthodox community. This differential access has a direct impact on couples' ability to plan families. First, in Judaism, the study of Talmud and of Jewish law has been constructed as a male sphere.[20] Even though there has been an immense growth of Torah study for Jewish women over the past thirty years, the study of Talmud and Jewish law remains largely the sphere of male expertise. This directly affects the differing ways Shimmy and Ayelet understand and interpret the meaning and authority of religious rulings.

The choice to bring their debate to "Shimmy's rabbi" creates an additional asymmetry as there is a gap between the prior knowledge and acquaintance the rabbi has with the couple. Whereas this particular rabbi knows Shimmy rather well, this may be the first time he met Shimmy's bride. The rabbi knows that Shimmy has been dating for a while and is excited to finally have children. We are not sure what he knows about Ayelet. He may think she seems a bit worried but will overcome her pre-motherhood jitters. Furthermore, because contraception issues are almost taboo, she may not know how and what to share with him. As such, he may not understand the intensity of her uncertainty, and she may not be comfortable sharing it with him. The alignment of two men in this encounter is particularly striking, as neither Shimmy nor the rabbi can experience pregnancy themselves. The embodied aspects of pregnancy linger in the room but are overruled and rendered invisible. Hence, in some cases, religious consultation is a sphere that permeates and reflects gendered power dynamics. In the Haredi community, where gendered separation is more enforced and sanctioned, it is more common for men to consult rabbis in the absence of their wives. This created a particular gendered asymmetry, as men debated contraception in the absence of the women who would bear the consequence of these conversations. Yet, even among Dati (Religious Zionists) who consulted rabbinic authorities together, rabbis were selected due to prior and/or personal acquaintance, usually with the male spouse, which propagated a different configuration of gendered inequality.[21]

But Shimmy and Ayelet's story did not end there. The disparities in their perceptions continued to grow as an unexpected neonatal tragedy challenged this process of decision-making. The birth of a sick and unresponsive child took the couple on a painful journey. They went through a cycle of mourning, crying, and blaming. Shimmy said: "We were optimistic and put ourselves into it. But we were also very realistic. We knew what all the options were, including the worst-case scenario that really ended up happening." Ayelet recounts the story:

> On Saturday night, Shimmy was out and I wanted to go to sleep. I went into Noa's room to cover her up with a blanket. [Ayelet breathes in and out.] I saw her hands were cold. So I covered her up with a blanket. It was dark. I came back ten minutes later to check on her and she was still cold. You have this second that you turn on the light and you already know what you are about to see. I screamed so loudly my neighbor called for an ambulance. I called Shimmy. I tried to resuscitate her. There was nothing left to do. The house filled up with people, and I remember sitting there on the sofa, knowing she was dead. Shimmy said we should say Tehillim [Psalms], and I remember screaming at him. At some point, everyone left and they took Noa. They took her and we stayed all alone.

Shimmy and Ayelet's story was not easy to hear. While conducting this research, I sat with many couples, never knowing ahead of time what curveballs life had sent their way. Shimmy and Ayelet's story stayed with me for a long time. In fact, I learned that for many couples, the effect and influence of the encounters with rabbis lasted long after the initial encounter. I was struck by the intensity of these effects and was intrigued to see the various strategies couples employed as they made sense of these encounters as time went on. Long after our conversation, I wondered: What does a couple think about a rabbinic ruling that ends up in such a tragedy? What does the weight of such a decision feel like when it is shared with others? Will they continue consulting with him and/or other rabbinic figures? Or is such a tragedy capable of creating a gap or a crack in this type of shared responsibility?

In Ayelet's case, it did. She recalled:

> That night I stopped taking [birth control] pills. I think that I wanted to hold on to life. But there was a deep change. Having Noa was a joint decision that I felt that I was being led to what is expected of me—from now on it was only my decision. Since then, I don't ask. I made the decisions and during that time . . . I remember my friend, who lived so close by I could hear her throwing up when she was pregnant. She went to a rabbi and he gave her three months to use contraception. I got so angry! How can a rabbi tell a young woman to get pregnant again in three months?

Ayelet decided to get pregnant immediately after this traumatic experience, but on her own terms. From that day on, she decided not to consult with anyone about her reproductive decisions. This transition reveals how even though Ayelet learned to engage in this practice and submit to religious rulings, it does not mean that the status of the religious ruling will stay untouched. Even more so, anger and critique turned Ayelet into an advocate against this contested mode of decision-making.

At this point in the interview, I realized Shimmy had become silent. I asked him to share his thoughts. Slowly, he shared how hard this was for him. Eventually, he explained, "When it came to making decisions, Ayelet's circle got smaller and smaller after Noa died. It started with keeping the rabbis out, and today I am also not included in this decision-making. Yes, it is her body, but what am I supposed to do when I want to have another child and she doesn't?" It was hard for him that it turned into a question that Ayelet decided by herself. Also, although this traumatic experience estranged Ayelet from rabbinic consultation, Shimmy stayed in a close relationship with his rabbi, who supported him through the hardships their life entailed. Whereas Ayelet's story is one in which she finds a path to disengage from rabbinic consultation, Shimmy reveals how shared responsibility creates a relationship in which the rabbi is constantly there for him. It is a special relationship that passionately guides him through this hardship. But it is more than that. It seems that sharing the responsibility with the rabbi gave him a voice in this decision, a voice that now seems lost. "I understand she pays the price for childbearing, but not being able to take part in the decision seems like complete male exclusion! No?" Ayelet smiles at him in agreement.

* * *

Rabbinic consultation serves multiple purposes. It provides an ethical compass during a time of uncertainty. In a community where sex and contraception are considered taboo, it provides a "kosher" space to consider taboo-like topics. Even though there are more and more public classes and guidebooks dedicated to the Jewish family, rabbinic consultation provides a private space for couples to voice their difficulties and search for new ethical horizons. Rabbinic consultation also provides authoritative mediation for couples who are struggling to coordinate their ethical compasses.

To be clear, by showcasing the ways Orthodox Jews engage with rabbinic authorities, I do not intend to cultivate a hierarchical model, positing one type as more "authoritative" than the other. On the contrary, if we take seriously Agrama's observation that religious authority is an expression of ethical agency,[22] we need to create new sensibilities for analyzing ethical agency in religious contexts.

At first glance, it may seem that "shopping around" displays the lowest level of following, while "navigating religious authority" reflects a midrange balance, culminating with "broad shoulders" as the highest and most pious degree of adherence. On the other hand, by applying the notion of religious consultation as an ethical language to the Jewish context, my ethnography questions whether the opposite is true. In other words, devotees cultivate a pious self through countless encounters with religious authorities, regardless of their adherence to religious rulings.[23]

My findings also reveal that dramatic life events challenge prior rulings. Traumatic experiences, like the death of a child or a miscarriage, have an especially powerful influence. Thus, notions of religious authority are worked out across a biographical trajectory, as traumatic experiences disrupt patterns of religious consultation and faith in religious authorities. These findings also push us to think about the ways in which authority fluctuates and changes in the lives of religious members as couples learn and unlearn the meaning(s) of religious knowledge. Sometimes, rabbinic mediation and guidance are exactly what they need. Sometimes, it is the opposite. It is not a black-and-white picture. The process changes from person to person, from couple to couple, and over the course of people's lives. I often found that while rabbinic consultation served as an ethical language when couples were first grappling with the need to talk about contraception, this did not mean they continued to obey these rulings forever. In contrast to other anthropologists who have overdetermined the power that rabbis hold over the lives of Orthodox men and women,[24] I argue that couples, just like Shimmy and Ayelet, often "unlearned" religious authority as they learned to challenge religious rulings based on their own lived realities. To be clear, challenging religious authorities did not make them want to leave Judaism, but it did push many of them to be critical of the religious obligations they had seemingly been committed to. Understanding what types of decisions are made amid these changing political and economic infrastructures requires examining how conflicting states of desire translate into creative frameworks of reproductive decision-making.

# 4

## Reorienting Decision-Making

One stormy winter evening, I entered the hall of a small community center on the outskirts of Jerusalem to attend a lecture entitled "Family Life and Jewish Law." As I walked in, my eyes latched onto a blue-eyed toddler playing on the floor, a big kippah (skullcap) on his head. "Is he yours?" I ask Adam, the man standing next to him. Adam, whom I had met at a previous lecture, smiles at me and answers, "No." A few seconds later, the child looks up and calls to him, "Daddy, can you help me?" Confused, I ask: "Is this a game"? Adam sighs and wholeheartedly replies: "He really isn't *mine*; he is God's child. We don't make children. We accept them as a blessing from God. Even if we wait for the right time to conceive, even as we learn how to wait and defer God's blessing, we must remember—they are not ours."

Adam, a modern-Orthodox father, offers a powerful critique of the local terminology used to portray kinship relationships between parents and their children. In Hebrew, the standard terms used to describe a child are "mine" (*sheli*) or "yours" (*shelach* or *shelcha*). These terms were rendered problematic, as they conceal the entire complexity of having a child. I understood that Adam was provoking me to rethink my own theory of kinship,[1] while transforming the exclusive relationship between children and parents so as to include God.

Adam's provocation reveals more than a terminological critique. Rather, it shows how the adoption of contraception ("even if we wait for the right time to conceive") is accompanied by a discursive strategy that renders parents as vehicles of God. In his reproductive narrative, I detected particular anxieties and paradoxes that were common among the couples I met. Reproduction has traditionally been a sphere of life in which God's presence is essential, and thus scientific knowledge threatens to displace God from the human-godly partnership.[2] As medical anthropologist Elizabeth Roberts has documented in her work among Catholics in Ecuador, reproduction was perceived as an assisted experience, and the valorization of science and individual autonomy "crosses God out of existence."[3] As growing economic, social, and bodily difficulties push parents like Adam to rethink their reproductive practices, I realized they needed to find a way to balance diverging desires and reproductive theologies. In this chapter, I use the concept "ethical choreographies" to describe this delicate coordination between the desires of the self, communal mores, and economic and vocational factors.

This conceptualization builds on Charis Thompson's work while taking on new meanings. In her groundbreaking ethnography *Making Parents: The Ontological Choreography of Reproductive Technologies*, Thompson introduces the concept of "ontological choreography," which refers to the "dynamic coordination of the technical, scientific, kinship, gender, emotional, legal, political, and financial aspects of ART [assisted reproductive technology] clinics."[4] Whereas Thompson focuses on the coordination process of elements that are generally considered parts of different ontological orders (e.g., part of self, society, nature), I develop this concept to capture how reproductive desires are coordinated to make an ethical life, both metaphorically and biologically.

I found that many couples, like Adam and his wife, Shelly, struggled to balance social, economic, and theological sensitivities within their reproductive narratives and practices. In what follows, I showcase the dynamics by which these multiple domains are coordinated to make an ethical decision. I draw on Thompson's work to show how ethical choreographies of decision-making are produced as couples reorient their reproductive desires and put forward creative grammars to mirror their ambivalent ethical stances.

I use the word "choreography" (the art of devising dances) to capture the ways these dynamics blend a fixed set of movements but also leave space for individualized performances of prescribed commandments and social expectations. This also hints at a circular movement that captures the temporality of ethical choreographies. As couples depart from straight and prescribed paths, new horizons become possible, but not without risk. The commandment to have children is not only about being a vessel to God's desire to populate the world. Straying away from a clear path of *Pru Urvu* (the first commandment requiring Jews to multiply) comes with a burden that has historically been compared to shedding blood. As Orthodox couples reorient their desires, they risk individual and collective promises of redemption. Ethical choreographies are not only a process of reorienting desires in the present moment but also entail a reorientation of one's futurity.

This chapter describes how these tensions result in unique reproductive models that form creative ethical choreographies that go beyond binary conceptualizations of planned/unplanned parenting. Instead, couples constructed a middle road, which I call "flexible decision-making," and built "gray zones" within which the categories of choice, desire, planning, and autonomy assume new connotations. For instance, some men and women chose, at one and the same time, to both defer and welcome pregnancies. Their narratives indicate that terms like "wanted" and "unwanted," or "planned" and "unplanned," are not necessarily mutually exclusive.

As part of their ethical choreographies, couples create subtle and fluid decision-making models. As reflected in Adam's narrative, while their own priorities pull the most weight, they also leave considerable room for the input of God, rabbinic authorities, their own bodies, and the voices of unborn souls. In parallel, they factored in and even welcomed the uncertainty variable, namely, that contraception might fail. These ethical choreographies allow couples to engage in contraception while coordinating practical considerations with theological sensitivities as they reorient their present and their future while striving to make an ethical life.

## Rethinking Reproduction

Today, it is rather intuitive to think of every child as either "planned" or "unplanned." Children are either a calculated choice of rational parents or a "mistake" made by irresponsible parents. But this has not always been the case. Buoyed by medical and technological progress, scholars of reproduction have shown how calculated and rational family planning has become a "project of modernity."[5] Anne Esacove describes how feminist scholars intentionally placed women's sexual behavior and the sphere of family planning in the realm of rational choice to challenge the idea of female reproductive behavior as "irrational" and "ignorant."[6]

While there may be many positive outcomes linked to placing the realm of reproduction in a rationalist paradigm,[7] this rationalist model has resulted in many underlying assumptions that have contributed to an inadequate picture of family planning. First, this mode of thought entails an assumption that reproduction, like any field of decision-making, is or should be driven by a calculated and fully intentional individual. Second, these underlying assumptions have created a dichotomous vocabulary in which terms like "wanted" and "unwanted" or "planned" and "unplanned" are treated as binary and exclusive.

In particular, the idea that an intentional, rational individual would choose not to take full control of his or her reproduction has become largely inconceivable, automatically turning any mode of ambivalence into a paradox. As anthropologist Heather Paxson put it, "It operates on the assumption that not only *can* people gain control of their lives, but that given certain knowledge they *will* make certain rational decisions and act accordingly."[8] Because of this stance, progressive media outlets, scholars, and policy makers laud such reproductive discretion, while condemning "accidental" pregnancies.[9] For example, a correlation is drawn between unplanned births and, say, child abuse, inhibited development, and a wide array of social ills.[10] Spearheading this "project," "Western" family planning experts and practitioners offer access to counselling, contraception, health education, and abortions.

However, when I was conducting my fieldwork, I realized that many of the people I met do not think about their reproductive desires in such black-and-white terms. As I collected reproductive stories, I often found it hard to decide whether the children some people had were a product of choice or not. While there were couples whose contraceptive strategies reflected binary thinking—either steadfast resistance or a general acceptance of "calculated" family planning, I also came across a third model, which I refer to as "flexible decision-making," where Orthodox couples engage in contraception while blurring the binary categories of choice, desire, and intentionality.

Challenging the common dichotomy between planned and unplanned parenting, I found that couples choose to resist and welcome pregnancies at one and the same time. The framework of flexible decision-making entails elements of adaptability, which create (almost) inconceivable situations in which children born to parents using birth control are still wanted and intended. Further, as reproductive decision-making is negotiated within and through many actors and systems of authoritative knowledge, this sort of paradigm also enables other factors, besides the immediate self or couple, to be involved in the decision-making, such as rabbis, professional advisers, the woman's own body, the souls of unborn children, and, of course, God. In what follows, I will explore these models of reproductive decision-making while highlighting the ethical choreographies they entail.

## Binary Conceptions

The first approach, shunning family planning techniques, was grounded in the idea that children are always a blessing from God, and thus, contraception should be kept to a bare minimum. Some of my interviewees espoused this approach from the outset of their marriage; others adopted it at a later stage. This view was quite common among couples from the low to middle socioeconomic status and among *baalei teshuva* (returnees).[11]

Liat (aged thirty), an educational consultant from a Mizrahi family, and Yoav (thirty-one), an Ashkenazi high school teacher, live in a national-Haredi settlement in northern Israel. At the time of the interview, they had four children and made it clear that birth control was never a viable option for them. As Liat related:

> After our first child, I was scared to get pregnant immediately. I would pray to God: "I am incapable of taking birth control, but I ask you to manage things the way they should be." I said this prayer for nine months while fully breastfeeding, so I didn't get pregnant. The second my period came back, I got pregnant. It was a nice break. Same thing happened after the second birth. After my second birth, I prayed to God that he would give me a child at a time when I could handle it best. And you know what? That is exactly how things worked out. You know, the third time I had a miscarriage. It wasn't easy, but everything is for the best. I really wasn't ready for another pregnancy.

This passage encapsulates the view that there is Divine Providence over all facets of reproduction. While hoping for a large family, Liat felt that she needed relief from parturiency in the months following childbirth. Since contraception is anathema to her, she conducted "private negotiations" with God, via prayer, over the length of these breaks.[12] At my encouragement, she elaborated on this approach:

> My friends use birth control. I have to say that it took me a while to accept it. In the beginning, I couldn't even hear of it. How can people do such a thing? Now I understand that for some couples it is important for their physical and emotional health. I have ruled out the option of [fam-

ily] planning. Come what may, we happily accept whatever God sends; it is a blessing.

Liat's husband Yoav, added with a smile: "The only thing we *plan* on doing is to adopt children at some point. In that respect, we are [engaged in] 'family planning.'"

According to this couple's family-building narrative, they have put themselves firmly in God's hands, for there is no such thing as an "unwanted pregnancy." You can pray for a break from childbearing, but God is fully in charge of reproduction and always knows what is best. Their narratives also entail an ethical judgment of those who choose to interfere in God's blessing, which they cannot "even hear of." Further, Liat and Yoav made it a point to show me that they are familiar with the modern term and practices of "family planning," but their reproductive strategy is portrayed as a critique of the contemporary family planning discourse, and they used the term intentionally in the atypical sense of building a large family.

Yet, as evident from Liat's description (and critique) of her friends, contraception is commonly used among observant Jews in Israel. In fact, already in the 1970s sociologist Rita Simon's study in Jerusalem showed that even though observant women were not using medical contraception, women who wanted to prevent or delay their pregnancies might postpone going to the mikvah until they reached their "safe period."[13] As mentioned previously, Jewish women tend to go the mikvah around the time of their fertility window, so this strategy reflects a premodern Jewish way to utilize the laws of purity, which effectively is similar to practicing the rhythm method or other low-tech family planning modes. These methods, as well as breastfeeding as a form of contraception, were still known and used when Michal Raucher conducted her research in Israel between 2009 and 2011.[14] While secular Jewish women primarily use the Pill and IUDs, as we have seen, Orthodox women today may use hormonal birth control but seldom insert an IUD or use condoms.[15]

Resonating with these studies, many of my interviewees who engaged in contraception described modern birth control as a "gift from heaven." This mode of thought was most prevalent among middle- and upper-class couples. A case in point is Evyatar (thirty-five), a Mizrahi high school teacher, and Ilana (thirty-three), an Ashkenazi physical therapist, who make their home in a Religious Zionist suburban community in southern Israel. During our interview, Ilana recounted:

> One of the mistakes I made was to have a child at the beginning of the year. That is the worst time to have a child. By the time I wanted to go back to work, my position was already taken by a substitute who did a great job. I learned that we would all have been better off if we had planned the timing of the pregnancy better. Why has God given us this ability if not to help make our lives easier?

Evyatar and Ilana perceive calculated family planning as a divine gift, which they were foolish not to have used earlier. They came around to this approach as their marriage progressed. "Learning from their mistakes," they reoriented their subsequent contraceptive decisions to take personal and professional factors into account. Further, as they timed reproduction to fit with Ilana's career, they put forward an ethical framework and language that reconstructed contraception as a gift from God.

Another couple, Hadas (thirty-five) and Avi (thirty-seven), both from Ashkenazi ultra-Orthodox backgrounds, held similar views, although their personal circumstances were rather different. Both teachers residing in a small town in southern Israel, it took four years for them to bring a child into the world. "You know," Hadas said, "even after the long process and grief of failing to have a baby, I think of how terrible it must be to have a baby when you don't have the energy for it. I would rather have no children than an unwanted one. God gave us the ability to choose; we must use it."

Like Ilana, Hadas perceives modern techniques and knowledge to "choose" as a blessing from God. Both couples came to this realization over an extended period during which their ethical choreographies reoriented conventional Jewish ideas to position birth control as divinely sanctioned. Whereas Ilana transformed birth control into a godly gift due to career needs, Hadas's close encounter with infertility solidified her powerful statement regarding the importance of intentionality. In contrast to the first approach where children are always desired, this second approach distinguishes between unwanted and wanted babies. Here the ability to have a child on a family's own terms is viewed as a positive possibility as human intentionality is rendered superior to Divine Providence.

## Leaving Space

The third approach, the most prevalent narrative I found, complicates the facile binary between total acceptance of "planned parenthood" and its rejection. According to this approach, God is an important agent, but other agents and modes of authoritative knowledge should be part of this ethical choreography. In these narratives, reproductive decision-making involves a constant juggle within a nexus of technical, scientific, gender, political, financial, and theological sensitivities. Because couples debated various factors, their accounts demonstrate the gray zones that blur the categories of both individual choice and intentionality as the exclusive ways to make reproductive decisions. Leah, a mother of seven from a national-Haredi background, explained:

> I went with my desires. Before every child, I couldn't wait any longer; I needed to have another one. Needed. And once again, I feel like having a couple more. They come to me at night and say, "Please." And they have names. And I see their faces. And I tell them, "I'm sorry, I can't; pick a different mother." And I cry and cry. I was dying to have another child. It's really hard for me. Hard to let my intellect decide. During the last pregnancy, I only told people when I was in my seventh month. I was scared of the responses from my family, from acquaintances. Stupid. Not

normal. I really hadn't spaced [the pregnancies]. But what can I do? My body wanted a child.

Leah focuses on her desire to have a child, and then another one, and another. These powerful desires led her to continue to have children without spacing them, even as her family and friends seem to object. Leah was not alone. I heard echoes of these parental desires again and again in my conversations with couples, particularly from women. Leah's desire to have seven births is negotiated vis-à-vis communal norms, especially those of her friends and her family. While she does not mention her spouse, I came across many women who also had to negotiate these desires with their husbands, who sometimes objected to these high-fertility practices. I vividly remember Ruchi, one ultra-Orthodox woman who was happily pregnant for the seventh time but was scared to tell her husband. She told me, "I knew he wouldn't be happy, so I prepared a whole romantic evening to break the news."[16]

Leah's struggle concluded with the following remark: "My body wanted a child." This sort of avowal was recurrent during my fieldwork, piquing my interest in deciphering the phrase. As I heard these multi-voiced and embodied self-discourses, I wondered what they could teach us about decision-making. What is the motivation behind this distinction between body and self? What is the difference between "I want" and "my body wants"? And in these situations, who decides whether or not to conceive?

I came across a persuasive explanation during an interview session with Merav (aged twenty-eight), a *baalat teshuva* (returnee), and Ari (thirty), who was brought up in a Religious Zionist family. Coping with three children under the age of five, they had just decided to use an IUD. Merav related:

Beforehand, I felt like I was repeatedly making decisions as if I am drunk. This time around I decided to go one step further [to avoid an unwanted pregnancy]. I chose an IUD because I felt that I needed to . . . make a real choice.... I need something permanent so that next time my body wants a child, I won't be blinded by it.

In using metaphors like "drunk" or "blinded" to describe her powerlessness, Merav gave voice to her sense that her earlier reproductive choices had been haphazard, that her body had basically "tricked" her and her husband into having another child. While both Leah and Merav describe their bodies as external actors that factor in their decision-making, only Merav viewed its sway negatively. Further, Merav's description renders bodily agency as inferior to "real choices," reflecting a perception of a hierarchy of intentionality in reproductive decision-making.

This hierarchy of intentionality became clearer as bodily agency was used to negotiate other types of authoritative knowledge. For example, Libby (thirty-seven), an ultra-Orthodox *baalat teshuva* art therapist, revealed how a traumatic experience transformed her outlook:

After my third child, I felt I needed to rest. We asked our rabbi, and he gave us permission to wait. I went to the doctor and put in an IUD, but it didn't stop hurting. At the hospital I found out that the IUD punctured my womb. At that very moment, I lost my faith in the medical system. We moved to a private hospital to remove the IUD, and that was the end of our visits to medical doctors. After the procedure, all I wanted to do was get pregnant. Thank God, there was no damage, and I got pregnant almost immediately. I was so thankful. I understood that trying to prevent pregnancies was wrong, that it was not God's plan. Therefore, I decided to never try birth control again. And that is how it was. I have seven children. My last birth was four years ago. I really can't think of having another kid and my body knows. So we aren't using birth control, but I know that I won't get pregnant again.

After three births, Libby turned to birth control. However, a painful experience with an IUD convinced the couple to put their faith in God and to shun the medical system.[17] Although they had permission from a rabbi to practice contraception, Libby and her husband interpreted a doctor's error as a holy message not to interfere in matters of procreation. This account reveals how bodily agency is used to disregard both medical knowledge and rabbinic authority. Michal Raucher has developed the term "reproductive agency" to capture how Haredi women do not turn to their rabbis, husbands, or doctors to make their decisions. After two or three successful pregnancies, their reproductive agency extends to all areas of reproduction.[18] Mirroring Raucher's findings, after seven children, Libby explained how her "body knows" that she does not want any more children and that she can rely on her body to avoid pregnancy. Putting aside the scientific probability (or not) of this, Libby's narrative reveals how contraception becomes closely linked with an unreliable medical system; the only system now on which she relies is her own body.

Another agent that surfaced frequently in these narratives was the voice of unborn souls, as Esther's narrative reflects. Esther was a thirty-eight-year-old National-Haredi housewife living in a West Bank settlement who told me the following:

> After my fourth child, I wanted to take a break. Hormones were driving me crazy, and just the thought of an IUD was unbearable. At the end, I found the perfect method of birth control—the diaphragm . . . it was a perfect fit for me. It had a 96 percent success rate. I didn't want another pregnancy, and I wanted to try to prevent another one. But if there really is a soul that wants to come down into this world, who am I to stop it?

According to Esther, modern statistics enabled her to make an optimal contraceptive choice. Since the method is not infallible, she claimed, other agents could take part in her decision. This reproductive approach undermines many of the binary categories we use when describing reproductive decision-making. Typically, a pregnancy that occurs despite the woman using a diaphragm would be considered "unintended." However, Esther constructed her utilization of birth control so that any outcome would be welcomed. By creating a gray zone, she blurred the binary distinction between wanted and unwanted pregnancies. This strategy allows for a situation in which a child born to a parent using birth control is still wanted, intended, and even planned.

The blurring of these categories resonates with medical anthropologist Don Seeman and colleagues' description of unintended pregnancy narratives among poor African American women in the southeastern United States.[19] These narratives highlight the tension between rational family planning discourse and the vernacular religious and moral ethos of pregnancy as a "blessing" or unplanned gift, and show how young and disadvantaged women may view pregnancy and unintended motherhood as opportunities to improve their lives. They reflect the "inadequacy of rational choice models that emphasize intentionality and planning,"[20] revealing a retrospective meaning-making discourse in a complex situation.

Yet, the gray zones I found were not used in retrospect but rather were considered informed decision-making from the outset. Some couples, like Sarah and Yitzchak, an ultra-Orthodox couple in their midthirties, established them for philosophical and existential reasons. As Yitzchak explained:

> Most religious leaders have been against this [i.e., contraception]. It's not just because of Jewish law. . . . You see, the moment a child is born is one of the special moments in my life. . . . I feel God's presence . . . ; there is some divine interference. . . . In medieval times, they didn't know what ovulation was and all these other things. Kids just arrived. When we moved to modern times, we have to ask ourselves "What is left of God?" The moment I know more and more, what is left for God in this world of knowledge? I think this is what lies at the heart of the objection to modern family planning.

In Yitzchak's estimation, the capacity to tinker with procreation has instigated a religious dilemma. Reproduction has traditionally been a sphere of life in which God's presence is rather tangible. Yet, modern knowledge and family planning are dislodging Providence from this realm. As God's crucial role in reproduction is undermined by scientific knowledge, Yitzchak and Sarah are confronted with an existential problem: "What is left of God in this world of knowledge?" At my urging, Yitzchak expanded on this matter:

> What is a human? What am I? When I say that "I am a decision of my parents," it contradicts the ability to see myself as a creature of God.... Nowadays, I have so much knowledge and I cannot shut my eyes. Shutting my eyes won't bring God into the picture. I have knowledge, and I also have a need for control. Should I refrain from taking charge just to leave space for God? There's really no solution. How do I make room for God so that when I sit with my kid, I can tell him that he is a child of God? I would like to live with the sense that I am not the creator of a child, even if I decide to push off the time of conception.

Modern knowledge and techniques are transforming childbirth from an act of God to a human endeavor. By clearing the way for, inter alia, calculated family planning, these developments also remove Providence from the equation. Nevertheless, Yitzchak and Sarah seek an ethical contraceptive route that preserves God's reign over procreation. By constructing a gray area, they grapple with an intellectual and existential paradox according to which both planned and unplanned babies are creatures of God.

* * *

As we have seen, social and structural transformations have contributed to an ideological and practical reorientation of reproduction. While scholars have documented widely how contraceptive decisions involve negotiating major social issues like femininity, masculinity, domestic roles, nationalism, and modernity,[21] I show how religious couples struggle with an additional challenge.[22] The transformation of childbirth from an act of God into a human endeavor engenders continuous ethical debates, which bring forward diverse, and often very creative, contraception strategies. The way contraception is viewed can lead to disparate, at times contradictory, behaviors as some couples shun modern knowledge and others fully accept it and even sanctify "calculated" family planning. Furthermore, the outlook espoused by my interlocuters was not necessarily set in stone under the *ḥuppah* (wedding canopy). Many couples modified their views in response to their life experiences, which forced them to make tough decisions.

One of the aspects of their approaches that I found most fascinating was that many couples built nuanced family planning models that were at variance with both the unbending rejection and the complete acceptance of twenty-first-century contraceptive methods. They constructed a middle road, which I call "flexible decision-making," and built gray zones within which the categories of choice, desire, planning, and autonomy assume new connotations. Flexible decision-making allows couples to postpone a pregnancy, but simultaneously to embrace it should it unexpectedly come to pass. Even more so, as reproductive decision-making is negotiated within and through many actors and systems of authoritative knowledge, this sort of paradigm also enables other factors, besides the immediate self/couple, to take part in the decision-making, such as God, rabbis, medical advisers, the woman's own body, and the souls of unborn children.

Flexible decision-making challenges two central assumptions that dominate scholarship on reproductive decisions: that decisions should be made by a calculated and fully intentional individual/couple, and that intentionality only appears in dichotomous notions (as terms like "wanted" and "unwanted" or "planned" "unplanned" illustrate). As they developed their ethical choreographies, couples formed fluid decision-making models that factored in and even welcomed contraception failure.

Could it be that this outlook is merely a creative strategy that couples use during this time of shifting social, cultural, and economic forces? In my estimation, this is not merely legerdemain aimed at preventing "unwanted children." I argue that these creative narratives contain unique modes of thought and ethical sensibilities. As couples struggle to take competing desires into account, their decision-making practices must be flexible enough to incorporate many (competing) factors in their ethical choreographies.

With so much at stake, it is clear why couples would linger in making these decisions and search for ways to challenge binary conceptions of decision-making. This also reflects what Homi Bhabha has called hybridity, which is characterized by creating an "in-between" space.[23] These ethical choreographies allow the couples I met to engage in contraception while coordinating technical, scientific, gender, political, financial, and theological sensitives as they reorient their present and their future to make an ethical life.

To understand these approaches to decision-making, it is necessary to emphasize not only what these choreographies entail but also what they omit. One consideration that was strikingly missing from these reproductive orientations was attention to environmental discourses. Over the past decade, scholars have documented how concerns about the planet are influencing family planning practices all over the world.[24] Even though, as anthropologist Katie Dow argues, "reproduction and environmentalism are both future oriented,"[25] in all of the courses and classes I attended, I never heard any mention of environmental considerations. During the course of my interviews, I met only one couple who had included environmental considerations in their decision-making—and they still ended up having four children.

In the Israeli context, religious communities are not known for their particular attention to environmental sensitivities.[26] While Jewish law offers many environmentally conscious theologies, these have largely been embraced by the progressive streams of Judaism. In fact, as we will see, in 2021 the Knesset introduced tax reforms aimed at decreasing the use of plastics. While these were formally introduced as environmental and health promotion amendments, they were criticized by Haredi members of the Knesset (MKs) as being anti-Haredi laws. Until this change, Haredi MKs supported high taxation on small plastic bottles but objected to raising the prices of large plastic bottles and sweet drinks, which are purchased by large families.[27] This critique reflects both state-minority tensions and inner communal notions that link environmental discourse with "secular" politics.

In the context of reproduction, therefore, it is not surprising that even though there have been advancements related to ecological thinking in Israeli society, these have not been widely adopted by Israel's Orthodox sectors. This reminds us that even as couples are reorienting their desires amid shifting social, economic, and political factors, the coordinates of our desires are always situated in particular discourses. Ethical choreographies do not entail a reorientation of everything. They reflect a situated sociocultural act of coordination, which highlights some factors as directives, while others are blurred in the margins. Ethical choreographies were also not the same for all but instead were highly stratified, as I show in the following chapter.

# 5

# Ending

> I would see queer as a commitment to an opening of what counts as a life worth living, or what Judith Butler might call a liveable life.
> —Sara Ahmed, *Queer Phenomenology: Orientations, Objects, Others*

During my fieldwork, many couples raised a painful question: "Is this it?" Sometimes this question surfaced at the end of our conversation, especially if the individuals were older and already had a relatively large family. At times, the question arrived earlier on, when they still had plenty of "biological" time, but wondered whether they should hold back on having more children.

As couples tried to find words to describe their family-building deliberations, they often referred to "straightening objects,"[1] like the family table or family photographs, which direct people to continue on certain (normative) desire lines. As we know, some lines lead to social recognition and privilege, while other lines are seen as "ways out of an ethical life, as deviations from the common good."[2] In what follows, I follow the straightening objects that appeared in the ethical choreographies of the couples I met. By highlighting the "work" these objects do, I pay attention to affective aspects of social pressure.[3] I demonstrate how these objects "call couples into line," but also highlight how couples learn to push back.

In doing so, I reveal a process of stratified reproduction that is based on social, economic, and religious capital.[4] While scholars of religious critique have demonstrated how religious elites behave as actors and leaders of resistance, my findings illustrate an opposite pattern.[5] Instead of disseminating this critique publicly, religious elites engage in private strategies of secrecy to diverge from norms without publicly contesting them. This hushed critique creates hidden power relations by which some people are empowered to nurture and reproduce, while others are not. Even though stratified reproduction is typically linked between social capital and *having* children, I flip the direction of causality. In my analysis, I show how religious elites critique reproductive norms secretly, creating a distinction between different subgroups of Orthodox communities, as it is specifically the newcomers, the returnees, who are less likely to critique communal norms. As the elite members secretly have fewer children or widen the breaks between pregnancies, they have more time to invest in parenting, focus on their own relationships, and direct more energy to work on professional advancement. Less privileged groups, and especially returnees who did not have the social capital necessary to secretly fail, end up with a burden that is often too heavy to carry.

Holding Back

Avi was a yeshiva student who had recently decided to study for a bachelor's degree by taking evening classes tailored for Haredim. Even though he loved to study, he felt that he could no longer devote his life to Torah study and had to find a way to supplement the salary that his wife provided. At the time of our interview Avi and his wife, Shifi, had six children, and they were not sure whether to have another one. After teaching at a seminary for over a decade, Shifi had recently become a vice-principal. She loved her new job, but it took much more time and effort than her previous teaching role. As the main breadwinner, she was not sure whether another baby would allow her to continue her work, which was challenging and satisfying, but also paid the bills.

As they grappled with this dilemma, both Avi and Shifi recalled particularly significant moments when they were forced to think about their choices. Shifi constantly referred to the pressure she felt when she went to the mikvah. As she would climb up the stairs, ascending from the water she had immersed in, she would stop and look at the prayer that was hanging on the wall: "And that God will bless me with children..." She now recalled, "I always used to read that prayer out loud. But now, I am not so sure that I want to. Sometimes I just whisper it, and sometimes I just skip that sentence. Each time I do something different." This prayer, then, works as a straightening device, as a reminder that when a woman steps out of the mikvah and goes back to being sexually active, one's desire is always directed toward children. A woman, thus, who leaves a mikvah without such a desire is reminded of this normative path, which she struggles with. Not being able to pray the same prayer as everyone else, or needing to alter the prayer, is a painful reflection of her own defiant desire, that just does not (or perhaps will not) align.

Avi also had such moments. He shared how Friday night dinners became the place where he was constantly reminded of the price he will pay for not having more children: "You know, I sit at the head of the table and look at Shifi. On both of the sides [of the table] three of our children sit. It is symmetrical and it is beautiful. On the one hand, it is a beautiful moment. I look at them as I hold the Kiddush cup, and I know that I am truly blessed. But, I know that there is more space at the table. Or at least there could be.... And I am holding the blessing back?" For Avi, sitting at the table serves as a straightening device. Resonating with Ahmed's analysis of tables, these objects make the "fantasy of a good life" visible. They also provide a source of discomfort and pain for those who deviate.

Years later, I recalled Avi's description when my husband and I bought a new table for our home. Even though there are five of us, we ordered a total of eight chairs so we could accommodate guests easily. As we sat down on the first Friday night, I looked at the three empty chairs and recalled Avi's description. I guess this is how he felt, I remember thinking: staring at empty chairs in the context of a Sabbath family dinner and wondering whether you should fill them with life. It also made me realize how powerful it feels to be called into line by an object. Even though the people I met were constantly navigating authoritative voices that intended to help them continue on the normative path, objects also served as straightening devices. While Shifi was reminded on a monthly basis and Avi was called into line on a weekly basis, each object, with its own temporality, was nudging them to stay on the large-family path at a particular ritualistic moment.

While Ahmed critiques heterosexual lines for (mis)leading toward a "promise of happiness," for the men and women I met, ethical choreographies were also linked to questions of righteousness. Shifi's inability to continue the traditional mikvah prayer and Avi's hesitation to hold back God's blessing remind us that their dilemmas fuse economic, bodily, and theological sensibilities that must be reoriented as they queer the perceived "righteous path." While Avi did not say so explicitly, when holding the Kiddush cup on Friday night, it is customary to allow the wine to spill a bit over the rim, to symbolize God's abundance and constant giving. I wonder whether that is what he meant when he referred to the wine.

Holding back (wine, seed, abundance) can be read as refusing a gift from God, which was a big theological challenge for many of the couples I met. I vividly remember how Ricki, a religious mother of five who was considering contraception, put it: "You see all these women who spend years going through IVF, just to have one child, and I should hold back on something that is handed to me on a platter?" In Israel, where IVF is easily available for all, children are perceived as gifts from God, even when they are born with the assistance of science. In a place where these children are heavily pursued, Ricki felt it was unthinkable to reject such a gift. Anthropological attention to gifts has long established that gifts come with gendered social obligations and debt.[6] But they can also serve as straightening devices. And what can be more heretical than holding back a gift from God?

As I listened closely, I found that there were also moments when objects helped couples defy the lines that they were supposed to follow. As our conversations moved on, Avi shared a reflection he had after coming home from a cousin's wedding. He explained that he was uncomfortable during all the family photographs. Each of his eight siblings posed for the camera, together with their growing families. He explained:

> At first, it made me feel bad. Baruchi has ten children. I watched as they stood together to make space for everyone in front of the camera. Then, it was Shoshi's turn. She has eight children even though she is younger than me. And, then it was our turn—and we only have six . . . but, you know what happened? The next morning I woke up and saw the picture of my family on the refrigerator. Shifi must have put it there before we went to sleep. I looked at the picture and thought—so that is it. And then it dawned on me. That is it. That is my family and it is beautiful.

Avi's reflection here is telling. While fighting social and familial models of a large family, Avi's narrative offers insight into a particular moment of transition. This moment is not part of a "life-changing" decision to change one's religious status (such as conversion or becoming Orthodox/un-Orthodox); instead, it presented a departure from one of the central parts of his religious path. A look at a photograph placed in an established mode of display (on the refrigerator),[7] which served as a straightening device the evening before, allows him to queer the expected path the next morning. When I use the word "queer" here, as elsewhere in this book, I mean to highlight moments when there is an "opening" of one's path, when new types of desire become part of one's horizon. In fact, the term "desire line" is a concept in landscape architecture originally used to capture an unplanned route or path; its formal definition is "an unplanned route or path (such as one worn into a grassy surface by repeated foot traffic) that is used by pedestrians in preference to or in the absence of a designated alternative (such as a paved pathway)."[8]

The spatial origin of this term is helpful here because it reminds us that in the absence of a designated path, people often create alternative paths, which leave marks on the grass they walk on. In our case, when the large-family path becomes unachievable, people find other ways to walk, while defying the "planned" and "normative" path, or *derech* (Hebrew for "path"). To an outsider, the choice to have only six children might not be seen as an act of defiance, but for Avi and Shifi this was not an easy decision. It put them on a different path than their siblings, one that reflected a change from their original course. Even though they had intended to walk on the "planned" path, they realized that to make a good family, they would need to walk on the grass. And, as Avi came to realize, this, too, was beautiful.

While Avi's reflections were linked to a feeling of beauty and completion, I also found deviation sometimes was linked to moments when desires visibly clashed. For example, I met Yaakov, an ultra-Orthodox yeshiva student and father of seven, at a coffee shop in Jerusalem, who told me:

> I had three girls first and loved playing with them. Then, I had a son. While the girls were young, I was happy to go on having children, but then my son started school and I started learning with him. I realized that if I want him to be able to be a learner, I need to learn daily with him. How could I do that if I have four more boys?

Yaakov's narrative reveals an intriguing phenomena. His decision to engage with birth control was based on his understanding that in order to educate his son(s) in the proper *derech* of the Torah, a way that would enable him to live up to the communal expectations of a boy, he would have to limit the number of children he had. Namely, Yaakov situated this decision in intracommunal gendered norms in which a father-son relationship was defined by the father's ability to teach his son to become a learned Jew. The commitment to biological reproduction stands in contrast to another kind of Jewish reproduction—the scholarly lineage.[9] This desire for himself and for the future of his son is a particular type of parental investment that he felt committed to. Thus, his decision to "hold back" was a product of two desires that could not be reconciled.

On the one hand, he wanted to continue the large-family "mission"; on the other, he also desired to be a good Orthodox parent who lives up to internalized communal expectations of Torah education. Thus, Yaakov's reorientation toward birth control is linked to particular communal norms of parenting, which become unachievable in the current state. Within this tough situation, Yaakov is searching for an alternative path while staying within Orthodox Judaism. The expression "off the *derech*" is often used to describe people who decide to leave the fold. But Yaakov is not leaving everything behind. On the contrary, it is his commitment to a particular form of Orthodox Judaism that pushes him to search for an alternative to the large-family path.

It is worth noting that there is a critical difference between Yaakov's choice here and Ahmed's phenomenology of desire. A comparison of the two reveals that there are different promises that linger at the end of particular paths. Happiness is not the promise that is directing Yaakov's life choices. Walking in the ways of the Torah is not driven *by* and *toward* happiness. In fact, the path *of* and *toward* righteousness has little to do with happiness. The way of the Torah is guided by duty, obligation, canon, tradition, merit, and God. This is the direction of a collective people who are all facing the same way. Yaakov, who is committed to continuing a scholarly lineage, must deviate from the large-family path in order to fulfill a competing desire and duty.

## Stratified Reproduction

Critiques of these reproductive ideals, though, were not available to all. As economic, social, bodily, and theological difficulties challenge Orthodox couples, I found that the strategies employed depended on their levels of literacy and their social status. I also found that, as in many other spheres of life, that critique was stratified. Critique was also often kept secret, a hushed strategy I mainly detected among well-situated and knowledgeable Orthodox couples. This is how Esti, an ultra-Orthodox

Bais Yaakov teacher, described the process of decision-making for herself and her husband, Dovid-Yisroel:

> As the wedding approached, Dovid-Yisroel told me he wanted to delay having children. I was very surprised. How could he not want children? He told me it was fine according to Jewish law, but I didn't believe him. I suggested we go to a rabbi. The rabbi said it is his obligation, and if he feels like he needs to wait, it is fine. I was so surprised. After we got married he would say to me, "Isn't it nice?" Having a quiet house. I really did enjoy it. But people started worrying. I had an accident right after I got married. I was fine, but people thought it had harmed my fertility. They would come over and say, "I am praying for you!" At the beginning, I felt bad not telling the truth, but after a few times I started to thank them politely. Their prayers will be helpful at some point.

Whereas most couples usually had children (or at least tried to have a child) before their first anniversary, some couples have recently started to use contraception before the birth of their first child. This practice has become common among modern-Orthodox Jews and is also slowly seeping in within various ultra-Orthodox communities. Dovid-Yisroel and Esti are an especially telling example of an ultra-Orthodox couple who must negotiate the divergence from this norm together. Interestingly, even after they receive rabbinic permission, the couple was uncomfortable sharing this decision with their families and friends. Because both of them are from prominent ultra-Orthodox families, everyone was sure they were having trouble conceiving. Indeed, I found that couples who decided to follow this trajectory were usually faced with family pressure and critique from friends.

During my fieldwork, I realized that I usually detected this hushed strategy among couples with a noticeable level of literacy as well as a relatively high social status. While this secrecy may have empowered these couples on a personal level, it also created a particular mode of stratification. I suggest the use of Shellee Colen's term "stratified reproduction" to make sense of this phenomenon.[10] In 1986, Colen introduced the term to describe the power relations by which some categories of people are empowered to nurture and reproduce, while others are unable to do so. In her study of West Indian nannies, Colen examines how these nannies perform physical and social reproductive labor to allow their female employers in New York City to go to work. She highlights how, rather paradoxically, the nannies allow their employers to have children and work, but their own reproductive capacities are diminished in a global economy that pushes them far from home. Colen's concept of stratified reproduction has been used to describe inequalities in the ability of people of different races, ethnicities, nationalities, classes, and genders to reproduce and raise their children amid structural inequalities.[11] Drawing on Colen's concept to explore the nexus of reproduction and stratification in a particular religious context, I argue that secrecy creates a distinction between the learned elite and the less knowledgeable members of Orthodox communities. In contrast to Colen's concept, which associates social capital with the ability to have children, I make an opposite argument. In this case, it is social and religious capital that enables couples *not* to have children.

This finding struck home during a course for bridal instructors I attended in Safed in northern Israel. An ultra-Orthodox *baalat teshuva* (returnee) named Michal, with seven children, shared some of her daily struggles with the class and then remarked: "I don't have any family to help me. I am an only child and even when my parents want to help ... they don't know how to handle all the kids ... and I can't send them to my parents or in-laws because their homes are not kosher." As I followed the conversation this remark inspired, I realized that, within Orthodox communities, nuclear families were deeply supported by their wider family networks. Sharing hand-me-downs and cooking meals together were just some examples of everyday assistance that families relied on. In large families, young and unmarried siblings routinely contributed to their married siblings' households. Also, within nuclear families, the

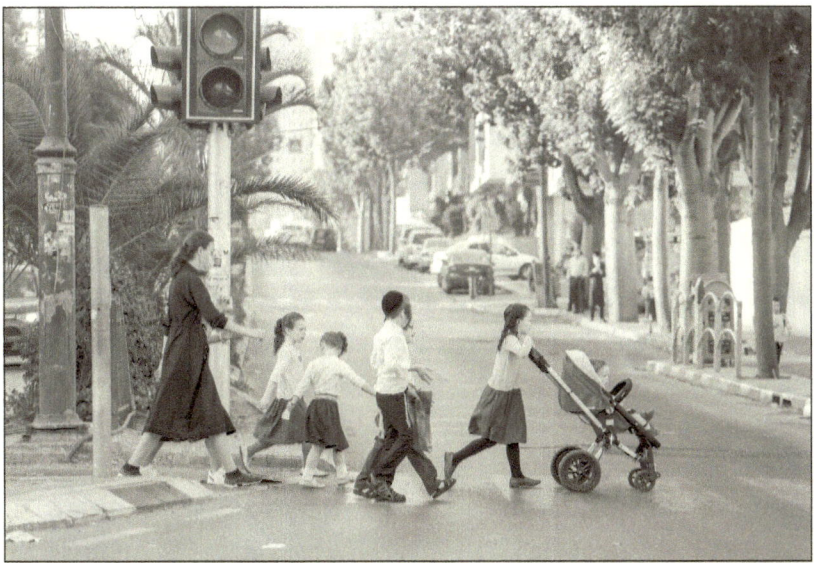

FIGURE 5.1. Haredi children attended by an older sister. Photo by Avishag Shaar-Yashuv.

oldest children, especially the oldest girls, would serve as "little mothers" from a very young age. When these girls grow up, they will also support their aunts who helped them when they were younger, creating an ongoing circle of familial assistance. Unfortunately, returnees did not have this type of help. Nevertheless, even though they seemed to be pursuing the almost unachievable ideal of large families in extremely difficult conditions, they did not want to let go of this promise.

As my intuition regarding this phenomenon grew, I raised this issue with one of the rabbis I interviewed. He smiled at me and said: "It is like chatting during prayer. Everyone does it but only the *baalei teshuva* will sit there silently. It takes a while for them to understand that Jewish law is not always black-and-white but many shades of gray." In other words, a direct outcome of these verbal taboos was that returnees were unlikely to understand which deviations were socially accepted.

In contrast to this, Esti and Dovid-Yisroel, whom I described earlier, are a great example of a couple from well-established families that had both the knowledge and the social positioning to decide to do something different. As mentioned previously, in the Talmud the religious obligation to procreate specifies only one or two children;[12] there is also an entire system of individual concerns that may be taken into consideration, such as physical and mental health, financial issues, and child welfare. Dovid-Yisroel grew up in the yeshiva world, and he knows the canonical sources well enough to understand that gray areas exist and that personal elements can be taken into consideration. Sadly, this knowledge was not available for everyone, and returnees did not understand the many shades of gray this performance entailed. Even if they were able to read between the lines, they did not have the social status or capital to take part in this performance until circumstances were truly onerous. They were too busy showing both themselves and their communities just how authentically pious they are. They did not have the social capital necessary to secretly fail in this highly-regarded mission. For them, taking an alternative *derech* or walking on the grass was just not an option.

This phenomenon raises many questions about the modes through which transformation occurs within religious communities. Even though transformation is not usually the focus of anthropological analysis,[13] scholars have tended to focus on elite and leading groups as the creators and perpetrators of communal norms.[14] For example, Nurit Stadler has shown how Haredi yeshiva students are the main forces of change, as they challenge the ideal of the Torah scholar. For those who face a changing economy together with growing expressions of feminism and modernity, the ideal of the fully committed Torah scholar cracks. Even though the yeshiva students embody the highest level of piety and would thus be expected to protect and maintain their piety privilege, Stadler shows how it is particularly the yeshiva students who challenge yeshiva piety and strive for a more "this-world-piety."[15] My findings, however, reveal the opposite. Whereas well-established, knowledgeable, and assertive religious members find ways to bypass the almost unachievable levels of fertility, a veil of secrecy leaves less privileged groups in the dark.

Ronit Irshai has described how the distinction between public Jewish law and rabbinic rulings given in private entails a selective concealment mechanism that primarily hurts disadvantaged populations.[16] Whereas Irshai has elaborated on this idea in terms of rabbinic decision-making, this project illustrates the social cost this type of strategy entails when it is further employed by religious elites. Because roughly 60 percent of returnees come from Mizrahi backgrounds, this finding also raises important insights regarding the inner categories of power that are reworked during this time of change. To be clear, I do not mean to claim that returnees follow communal norms blindly. Yet, the elite's hushed critiques create a double standard as it is their public reproductive discourses and practices that set communal standards.

I suggest that the divergence from the scholarship on religious critique is linked to the sensitivity of the topic at hand. When Orthodox members critique "public" norms like participation in the workforce, their critique cannot be hidden.[17] As yeshiva students wish to leave the yeshiva to pursue academic studies and advance professionally, they must critique their leaders publicly in order to receive public recognition and approval.[18] However, if a couple does not have a child within a year of marriage, no one will know what the reason is unless they choose to share their motivation with their community. Private matters, thus, can enable more room for flexibility and secrecy, which is always a double-edged sword. My findings reveal that during a time of uncertainty regarding reproductive norms, religious elites act secretly.

These strategies do not only reflect social inequalities, they deepen them. Resonating with the findings of social theorists on moments of social transformation, social stratification often finds creative ways to replicate preexisting modes of power. When I began this project, I thought I would find race and ethnicity as leading forces of inequality among my research participants. I was surprised to find that high levels of piety and religious elitism would be the main forces behind stratified reproduction. But, as the elite members quietly lower the number of children they have or widen the gap after each birth, they give themselves more opportunities to focus on their parenting and, ultimately, on the socialization of the next generation. They also allow themselves more time to focus on deepening their own relationships and to invest more time and effort in personal and professional advancement. This finding begs us to take a closer look at the ways in which reproductive practices intersect with other systems of power, such as religious social capital. As explored in the next section, not having the time and energy to do so can have far-reaching implications.

## Back to Shlomo and Miriam

I vividly remember sitting on the cold stone steps outside of Shlomo and Miriam's house after they shared their reproductive story with me. I just could not get into the car and drive home. I was too sad. I was surprised at how sad their story made me. I had heard couples talk about miscarriages, cry about children dying during childbirth or a few months after, and here I was, sitting on the stone steps, after a couple shared their "regular" family difficulties with me.

Something about Shlomo and Miriam's story really hit me. They had constantly tried to smile as they shared with me their struggles to make an ethical life for themselves and for their children. They had three beautiful children, who all peeked at me from the family photographs that covered the fridge in their apartment. But I could not shake off the sadness that lingered, even after I left their home. With three young children, they were constantly asking the questions I presented at the beginning of this book: "Who is first? My husband? My children? The house? Work? My body? Who is first?" As they struggled to reconcile their own ethical choreography, they reached a breaking point. As Shlomo told me:

We are not breathing. The Sabbath has turned into a nightmare. You cannot even imagine. It is really hard. And do you know what? We have changed. Sometimes, I think that on the long summer days of Shabbat I should just take the kids to the pool . . . just to get them out.[19] We have changed, but the only thing that can't change is the fact that you have children. You can get a divorce if you want, but your kids will not disappear. . . . I think that we both feel that if we had a choice, if we knew then what we know now, I think we would have waited more before having our first child, and we wouldn't have rushed so quickly to have our third.

Shlomo pauses. He eventually looks up and continues, "We have decided that at this point we don't want to add any more variables. We need to love what there is."

Sometimes the timing of an interview can be very important. Interviewing a couple at the end of August in Israel, where there is no subsidized childcare during July and August, certainly seemed to reveal a higher level of frustration for parents. Shlomo shared with me how their difficulties pushed him to rethink some of the basic rules of the Sabbath. His contemplating taking the children to the pool on the Sabbath, a sin in his community, reveals the extent of their difficulties, which embody a clash between desires that do not seem to be easily reconciled. In the face of these difficulties, they had recently decided to change their reproductive strategy, and at the time of our interview, Miriam already had an appointment to have an IUD inserted.

But even though I kept telling myself that Shlomo and Miriam sounded so tired because it was August, something about their story indicated that there was more. Two years later, I heard that they had separated. I wanted to pick up the phone and ask them what had happened, but the truth is that I felt like I already knew. I knew that the cracks were just too much for them. In fact, I went back to my transcripts and read Shlomo's words again: "You can decide to get a divorce, but your kids will not disappear." I guess a part of them already knew what was coming. This is not to say that divorce is always bad, but I felt that I had watched the unraveling of a family dream, and it hurt. Even though they decided to "love what there is," this, too, proved too difficult at this moment in time. In addition to being pressed to let go of the large-family desire, they ended up letting go of their promises to each other. This painful understanding pushed me to wonder whether this outcome could have been different if only they had chosen to diverge from social norms. Would they still be married if they had decided to use birth control before they had their first child, as Esti and Dovid-Yisroel had been able to?

Esti and Dovid-Yisroel's conviction to wait before having their first child was relatively uncommon among the couples I spoke to. I recalled how many couples shared the excitement of getting pregnant without fully comprehending what this entailed, often without bringing up the topic of contraception at all. I will always remember my chat with Ruchi, as we both sat on a wooden bench as her three young children played in a small park behind her home. We had met a few times before, but this time, she mentioned an additional detail that had not surfaced previously. As she told me about the birth of her first daughter, Yael, she got angry and said: "Yael is a product of a panel." Filling in the gaps for me, she recalled how right before her marriage she had attended a day of learning, which included one panel on having children. "Even though Judaism is all about rabbis disagreeing," she explained, "they all seemed to agree about having kids. While there were three rabbinic figures on the panel who were talking about the various halachic aspects of family life, they all seemed to agree that there is never a good reason to delay the birth of a first child unless the mother or child are in danger." Ruchi pointed at the little girl who was swinging with her younger sister on a squeaking yellow seesaw, and repeated what she had already said: "Yael is a product of that panel!" As I digested Ruchi's critical take on the backstory of her first child, I imagined that the rabbis on the panel, just like many other educators who pushed couples toward the large-family path, never heard these stories. They had no idea how much power their words had. I also thought about the price of walking down a path that seemed to be well-trodden but was, in reality, becoming harder to continue. Cultivating ideals that are framed as timeless does not promise a manageable life. On the contrary, it runs the risk of fostering a commitment that winds up crushed in the sea of life.

Following Miriam and Shlomo's divorce, I took a look at national divorce rates. Compared with the OECD average divorce rate of 1.7 per 1,000 people in 2020, Israel has a similar rate of 1.8 per 1,000.[20] Within the Israeli Jewish population, divorce rates have been on the rise, doubling since 1970. Among Jewish denominations, whereas divorce rates among religious (Dati) couples have remained stable (11 percent), divorce rates among Haredi Jews have doubled in recent years (from 3.7 percent to 6.6 percent).[21] It seemed like Shlomo and Miriam's situation reflected a growing trend, one that can also be detected in the number of classes and initiatives devoted to strengthening the Jewish family, described earlier in this book. To be clear, this ethnographic study cannot (and did not set out to) identify a causal link between shifting state policies and ultra-Orthodox divorce rates. Nevertheless, studying Orthodox reproduction in the aftermath of vast policy changes pushes us to study their ripple effects.

* * *

Orthodox Judaism, as Yaakov Katz, put it, is a modern phenomenon.[22] While it frames itself as following age-old practices and ideologies, Orthodoxy is sustained and shaped by particular nation-states and public policies. For years, Orthodox Judaism has flourished in Israel's pronatalist system, but as these reproductive logics transform, it has become much harder to maintain large-family norms. Although, as I have described, straightening objects serve as constant reminders for all, some people are able to queer them. I have shown how couples reorient their family desires either when their desires collide or when they have enough social capital to imagine new horizons for gender, intimacy, family, and parenting. Amid a moment of shifting state infrastructures,

Haredi men and women struggle to mend the gaps by searching for alternative spaces in which to learn and debate about contraception. Yet, as I have shown, these shifting policies do not have an equal effect on everyone. Instead, these changes link on to preexisting systems of hierarchies, in this case, religious-based social capital, which is deepened and reproduced during these moments of transformation.

Most of the couples I met frame their struggles as personal, often referring to seeking psychological help to mediate their personal difficulties.[23] However, I highlight the structural shifts that have forced couples to navigate difficult dilemmas. Indeed, most of the people I met agreed that having a large family was an important ideal, one they wished to continue, if only they could. With Israel's new public policies, their desire to have a large family was put into direct conflict with other desires such as ensuring a good life for one's children, having an intimate relationship with one's spouse, and, as many of the parents I interviewed put it, "just breathing." Taken altogether, this book demonstrates how Orthodox desires and their discontents are reshaped at the intersection of reproduction, religion, and politics, even in the most traditional settings.

# Coda

As I write the coda to this book, there has been a shift in Israeli politics.[1] After fifteen years of Benjamin Netanyahu's reign over Israeli politics, new alliances came forward, positioning Naphtali Bennet as prime minister, with a newly assembled coalition pushing for a different agenda. Even though Bennet stated that the new focus of the freshly formed government is to heal inner conflicts, on July 7, 2021, Avigdor Lieberman, the newly elected minister of finance, announced a dramatic change in Israel's public support of childcare. Whereas, in the past, the criterion for state funding for childcare was based on economic status, the new model focused on the professional or educational status of both parents. Developed to support the incorporation of young parents in the workforce, this new policy offered financial support to parents who work at least half-time or are studying to acquire a profession. While this might seem to be a minor bureaucratic change, it was closely linked to the economic and reproductive logics described in this book. Namely, the new policy would primarily disadvantage Haredi families, where fathers mostly study in a yeshiva and do not typically participate in the workforce. Until now, as long as the Haredi mother worked (at least part-time), Haredi families were eligible for state funding, whereas in the new scheme, this would no longer be the case. This policy change would save the state 400 million shekels, but it would affect the lives of twenty-one thousand Haredi children and their parents, who currently rely on this funding.

Haredim in Israel were furious. While Lieberman stated that this new "order or priority" would "put a stop to the continuous distortion in Israel where the working public is discriminated against,"[2] Haredim perceived this "daycare decree" as evil, while comparing Lieberman to many of the historical "evil leaders," such as Pharaoh. In particular, these parallels draw links between Pharoah's demographic concerns regarding Jewish reproduction ("He will be multiplied and he will be called war" [Exodus 1:10]) and Israel's current affairs. As Haredi MK Litzman stated: "Lieberman is implementing a policy of '*pen tirbe*' of the evil government headed by Bennet and Lapid, which goes against the Haredim and the Jewish tradition. This is a direct and concerted act against Haredi families, born from disgust and hate of married yeshiva students and large families."[3] Linked to biblical narratives of reproductive governance, referred to vernacularly as *pen tirbe* ("he will be multiplied"), this critique reflects competing ideas of what supporting a family looks like. Haredi MKs also mentioned that Lieberman is influenced by his Russian background, in which "he was educated against religion." They claimed that he took the first possible moment to make this change, as he took on a new role as minister of finance in the newly formed government where Haredi MKs were not part of the coalition.

Haredi families and childcare providers immediately appealed to Israel's high court, demanding that it stop or at least postpone this drastic policy change. These appeals also drew support from the Religious Zionist group known as *toratam umanutam* (Torah scholars with no other profession), which put pressure on the religious MKs who are still part of the coalition to stop this change, since many Religious Zionist men study full-time, too. To cut a long story short, on January 12, 2022, Israel's high court ruled that the timing of this policy change was problematic and did not leave parents enough time to prepare for the year ahead. The court ruled that this abrupt policy change would end up harming children and, thus, delayed its start date.[4]

The battle against the "day care decree" did not come out of nowhere. While these thorny tensions had been brewing for years, they picked up speed amid the COVID-19 pandemic. Haredi Jews accounted for 40 to 60 percent of all coronavirus patients at four of Israel's main hospitals, even though they make up only 12 percent of Israel's population.[5] In response to the disproportionate effects of COVID-19 on Haredim, a wave of public critique swept over Israeli media, where pictures of Haredi Jews defying public health guidelines began to appear daily. This critique was reciprocated and kindled Haredi suspicions of the "true intention" behind the decision to shut down religious seminaries and synagogues during the pandemic, reflecting a lament of many Haredim that secular Jews are allowed to gather to protest, but Haredim are not permitted to gather to pray, mourn, study, or celebrate.

In a study I conducted with two colleagues, Ayelet Baram-Tsabari and Yael Rozenblum, we found that when Haredi participants were asked what they thought about the Ministry of Health's decision to close all schools, universities, and religious seminaries, most respondents agreed that the decision to close all schools and universities was correct (94.9 percent), but only 23.2 percent agreed with the decision to close religious seminaries.[6] This points to the disparity between how public health guidelines and regulations are perceived in the context of general education as compared with how guidelines should be applied in a religious context, reflecting many of the tensions described in this book.[7]

In the context of the COVID-19 pandemic, even though the comparison between schools and religious seminaries was fairly intuitive for Israeli policy makers and reporters, from a Haredi perspective the government decision to close all religious seminaries was perceived as shutting down the heart of Jewish life. The constant comparison between religious seminaries and schools reflected how public policy makers and commentators ignore aspects of Jewish life that are essential, according to Haredi frameworks. As Rivka, one of the participants in our study, said: "Religious seminaries and the army are the same. . . . It is a home and there is no reason to send them home. They can maintain the guidelines there!" For Rivka, the comparison between the army and religious seminaries is the "correct" comparison, one that equates the importance of studying Torah with the army as different ways of maintaining a Jewish state. While the comparison to the army may come as a surprise, it is actually common among Haredim. Haredim are constantly criticized for their exemption from compulsory military service, which also challenges their fulfillment of the duties of all Israeli citizens. The frequent comparison between army and Torah study typically supports Haredi logic that Torah study spiritually sustains Israeli society.[8]

As life gradually shifted to a "new normal" after the most restricted period of the COVID-19 pandemic, these thorny state-religion tensions were rekindled with the formation of the new government, which was the first time Haredi MKs were out of the government in decades. The outrage that emerged with the introduction of the "day care decree" was thus only a tiny part of the fury that emerged with the new coalition. But, as I have argued in this book, this is not just a product of a new game of musical chairs in the Knesset. Amid growing demographic anxieties, Haredi Jews have constantly been singled out in public policy, especially in the context of reproduction. Mirroring age-old questions about Jewish belonging and competing models of citizenship, these are mere reminders of the powerful pronatalist logic that underlines Israeli biopolitics. With the shift from a desire to reproduce Jews to maintain a Jewish majority, a new set of desires drive Israel's agenda today. With the anticipated growth of the Haredi population characterized by low levels of secular education and minimal participation in the workforce and the army, together with an ambivalent relation with what is perceived as the "secular" state, the growth of the Haredi population ushered in new forms of reproductive governance aimed at managing and reducing the growth of Israel's religious sectors, a transition that lies at the heart of this book.

\* \* \*

This is a book about the ways our most intimate desires are shaped by state policy. While desire has long occupied the thoughts of philosophers and psychoanalysts, ethnographers do not tend to focus on desire as an object of analysis.[9] Thinking about desire requires making unusual theoretical connections, however unorthodox they might seem. To study the reorientation of Orthodox desire, I use Sara Ahmed's work as a theoretical compass. Even though her queer phenomenology was developed in a vastly different context, I draw on Ahmed's ideas to highlight the experiences of disorientation among Orthodox Jews as they rethink some of their most basic desires. As neoliberal desires to cultivate a high-income and high-tech nation merge with particular Jewish demographic anxieties, cracks have appeared in one of the most important ideals of Orthodox Jews—making a large Jewish family. This book captures how cracks in religious convictions engender a painful process of orientation amid rapid structural change emerging from shrinking public support, feminism, and new ideals of romance, intimacy, and parenting. I have charted how these changes create difficult ethical dilemmas that push couples to make hard decisions, as they debate between following the large-family path and their desire to offer their children (and themselves) a good life. Paying close attention to dilemmas, ambivalences, and failure, I have aimed to show how life can become disoriented when one's path becomes obscure. When one's basic orientation of what is left, right, up, and down becomes unclear. When the ground one stand on shifts. When the directionality of one's path becomes uncertain.

Jews are meant to follow the *derech* of the Torah. They are meant to "walk in his ways" (Deuteronomy 28:9) by following the rules of halacha, which literally means "to walk." To make a righteous life is to walk on a particular path. And the pressure to "stay in line" is paved by straightening objects and human agents who nudge people to continue the normative walk. But, even though straying from the path is risky, the men and women I spoke with found ways to cultivate new desires. They found a "kosher" language to voice their debates. They went to speak to their rabbis, who served as ethical compasses during a time of uncertainty. They crafted unique modes of reproductive decision-making and creatively engaged with modern contraception. Torn between conflicting desires, they crafted particular ethical choreographies through which technical, scientific, gender, political, financial, and theological sensitives are coordinated. Straying from the path is risky, and still, desire lines create new pathways.

This ethnographic account of the reorientation of desire offers an empirical depiction of shifting desires. Taking Ahmed's phenomenology as a starting point, this account showcases how desires are formed and resisted in everyday life. By pointing to the sociopolitical shifts in Israel's state of desire, I highlight some of the forces that shape the path, or perhaps the ground the path lays upon. In doing so, I disrupt the "fantasy of natural orientation" by historicizing the ideal of the large Jewish family.[10] This book offers a new approach for scholars interested in the social construction of desire. To develop the analysis of desire, I offer a few conceptual tools—such as ethical compasses, horizons, and choreographies, that offer overlapping spatial and temporal imaginaries to illuminate how desires are shaped and reoriented amid shifting discourses and public policies. In this way, this ethnography also stresses the importance of studying how individual and national desires are intertwined. Thus, the "state of desire," the title of this book, refers to a particular state that has continuously acted to shape the most intimate desires of its citizens, but also serves as an analytical tool to be used to study the sociopolitical conditionings of desire anywhere.

When I talk about my work with a nonanthropological audience, people are often uneasy about the emphasis I tend to put on the ways we are all influenced by the social, political, and economic structures in which we live. People often prefer psychological approaches that give more space to desires that come from "within." But sociological and anthropological research point to the specific ways we are shaped by particular cultural scripts and state infrastructures. From Émile Durkheim's attention to the social aspects of suicide to Pierre Bourdieu's analysis of class-based taste, social theorists have powerfully shown how culture goes deeper than we think. My work joins this ongoing attempt to expose how culture shapes us, but I also pay close attention to how people push back.

There is a potential risk in exploring these questions in the context of Orthodox life. Framed as maintaining an age-old way of life, Haredim are often depicted as "stuck in the past" or overly obedient to what is perceived as the authentic version of Judaism. It is for this reason that much of the scholarship exploring Orthodox agency focuses on people who decided to leave the fold (go off the *derech*).[11] However, the prevalence of debates and dilemmas that occur in the everyday lives of people who live within the *derech*, showcased in this volume, reveals that there are multiple paths to walk within Orthodox Judaism.

Going beyond the Protestant-inspired tendency to focus on belief, I have shown how doubt is also part of religious life. I argue that there are all kinds of ways that religious subjects navigate lived experience versus some kind of ideal, whether canonical texts or a family picture hanging on the fridge. By charting how reproductive theologies are built from the ground, my analysis accounts for theologies that emerge from lived experience. As the telos of large families is threatened, men and women form fresh repro-theologies that reshape concepts such as religious obligation and its limits. In showcasing these debates, this book disrupts and challenges anthropological readings of religious subjectivity as a form of submission. While scholars of religion have offered detailed accounts of how religious doubt leads to "heresy" and abandonment of faith,[12] this book shows how Orthodox desires and convictions concerning reproduction are reconfigured from within when confronted with social change.

This study also questions one of the main understandings regarding social change in religious contexts. Scholars have constantly demonstrated how religious elites act as agents of reformation, but my findings indicate the opposite. I have found that during a time of uncertainty, religious elites act secretly. As elite members lower the number of children they have, devote more time to deepening their relationships, and invest in their parenting and, ultimately, in the socialization of the next generation, they leave less privileged groups struggling to live up to almost unachievable ideals. Not only does this analysis offer new ways to think about how stratified reproduction is context-specific, but I also argue that we must look at the ways reproductive dynamics are linked to other social inequalities within religious communities and well beyond.

Even though religion has been often pushed to the sideline in reproductive politics scholarship (which has focused more heavily on various forms of inequality), I argue here that religion matters in studies of the state. As I write these sentences, the US Supreme Court has voted to overturn *Roe v. Wade*, a landmark legal ruling that has guaranteed federal constitutional protections of abortion rights since 1973. The Evangelical forces that shaped this moment offer a clear reminder of how religion and the state cannot truly be understood separately, especially in the context of reproduction. Drawing parallels between these two vastly different contexts, though, begs us to looks for commonalities and disparities. How do particular forms of state-religion relationality inform reproductive politics? How do notions of religiosity and righteousness affect the "secular" court and systems of public policy? And what forms of inequality do these forces put forward? We need to do better at understanding these dynamics.

Further, while scholars of religion and race are rarely in conversation, recent works have pushed for more analysis of the race-religion interplay.[13] My work here builds on these insights by providing a vivid example of when and how religion can become raced. Similarly to the way Su'ad Abdul Khabeer describes how Islam in the United States is often coded as "Black," my analysis has been built on an understanding that Haredim are often racialized in the Israeli context.[14] I have shown here how Israel's reproductive governance is also linked to racialized imaginations of religion that reflect tensions regarding the desire for a particular "Jewish state."[15] This finding resonates with Saba Mahmood's argument that modern secular governance entails "fundamental shifts in conceptions of self, time, space, ethics and morality, as well as a reorganization of social, political and religious life."[16] Reproduction is but one example of the overlap between epistemic, political, and social imaginaries of the liberal "secular" state as it tasks itself with the management of family life. Ethnographic attention to the nexus of demography, race, and religion is critical for understanding these overlapping systems of oppression.

Methodologically, I hope that a significant contribution of this work is its effort to incorporate male perspectives into a field that is dominated by women's experiences.[17] This book not only offers a rebalancing act but also demonstrates how reproductive politics shape male and female desire, albeit in different ways. This intervention has an additional benefit in the context of Jewish studies, which has been dominated by a gendered distinction between studying men in the yeshiva and women at home. By utilizing couple interviews, this study gives voice to both female and male desires, challenging hegemonic depictions of Jewish femininity and masculinity.

Finally, cultural analysis of reproduction has focused primarily on new reproductive technologies. As innovations have been introduced in the field of reproductive biomedicine, each new development has garnered vast attention, especially from medical anthropologists and feminist, legal, and science and technology scholars.[18] Yet, I am concerned with the ways the study of contraception has been pushed aside within reproduction studies. Feminist scholars have repeatedly shown how contraception is often used as a vehicle for biopolitics, and thus closely linked to projects of political governance. This state interest in managing populations does not seem to be changing. In addition, even though contraception has been around for as long as we can remember and developed rapidly since the invention of the Pill in 1960, we also still lack a nuanced understanding of how people engage with contraception. For example, this work challenges the common dichotomies between planned/unplanned and wanted/unwanted children. This finding advances the work of other scholars who have pointed to the inadequacy of rational choice models that overly focus on intentionality and planning. Amid a global ecological disaster, grasping a better understanding of how people make decisions amid ethical uncertainty seems more urgent than ever.

I am constantly asked about the future. With an eye to the larger historical stakes of intervening in personal life, I am very anxious about state attempts to control, shape, and manage population in Israel and elsewhere. I hope this book offers another reminder of how violent public policies can be, even when their intentions are seemingly positive. This ethnography shows how demographic forecasts bring forward invasive modes of sovereignty that affect the most basic desires of citizens, but it also reveals how people dare to walk unconventional paths, even in the most traditional settings. Amid shifting modes of reproductive governance, I have seen how creative people become as they navigate the delicate balance between state policy and individual desire, an ethical choreography we all dance in different ways.

ACKNOWLEDGMENTS

Ethnography is only possible when people let you in. I am truly grateful to the many couples who shared their most intimate struggles with me. Even though I cannot thank you all by name, I hope you can hear the echoes of your stories in this ethnography.

Writing this book would never have been possible without the help and support of many colleagues. First and foremost, I want to thank my academic mentor, Nurit Stadler. I am grateful to you for introducing me to the beauty of anthropology of religion. Thank you for shaping my intellectual interests and providing tools to pursue them. Your wisdom, intellectualism, and persistence on both methodology and theory shape every project I undertake. Thank you for inviting me into the family and for always being there.

Moving from Hebrew University to the University of Cambridge adds a further list of people who have made me feel at home in a new environment. First, thank you to Yael Navaro for pushing me harder than I could ever have imagined. Special thanks are also due to James Laidlaw, Joel Robbins, and Matt Candea. I am also grateful to Sarah Franklin for the constant gift of her mentorship. Thank you for being a brilliant source of wisdom and feminist spirit and for insisting I write this book as simply as possible. I also owe a big thank-you to members of the ReproSoc team, especially Katie Dow, Marcin Smietana, Noémie Merleau-Ponty, Lucy Van de Wiel, and Robert Pralat. My thanks also go to Edward Kessler, Esther-Miriam Wagner, and Emma Harris for inviting me to become part of the Woolf Institute, which turned into another intellectual home for me. Newnham College has been an additional source of support—special thanks to principal Alison

Rose, Liba Taub, Emma Mawdsley, as well as Harriet Truscott for her brilliant support.

My thoughts were also shaped by several opportunities to present portions of this book, where many insights emerged through countless discussions, debates, and lively critical questioning. These include the Oxford Institute for Contemporary and Modern Judaism; the Jewish studies program at the Sorbonne; the Department of Jewish Studies at Fordham University; the Centre for Research in the Arts, Social Sciences and Humanities at the University of Cambridge; the Belfer Center for Science and International Affairs at the Harvard Kennedy School; the Department of Demography at the Université Catholique de Louvain; the Religions and Theology Department at the University of Manchester; and the Anthropology Department at École Pratique des Hautes Études.

This book is also a product of countless conversations with more people than I can name here. Thanks are especially due to Tali Artman, Orit Avishai, Daphna Birenbaum-Carmeli, Noga Buber-Ben David, Morgan Clarke, Lynn Davidman, Theo Dunkelgrün, Jodi Eichler-Levine, Tamar Elor, Sami Everett, Rachel Feldman, Adam Ferziger, Sylvia Fishman Barack, Michal Frenkel, Miri Freud-Kandel, Katie Gaddini, Simon Goldhill, Shlomo Guzmen-Carmeli, Yael Hashiloni-Dolev, Marcia Inhorn, Ronit Irshai, Tsipy Ivry, Michal Kravel-Tovi, Nissim Leon, Severine Mathieu, Ashira Menashe, Rivka Neriya Ben-Schahar, Sophie Nizard, Vanessa Ochs, Barbara Okun, Yaron Peleg, Don Seeman, Sertaç Sehlikoglu, Yang Shen, Shaul Stampfer, Michal Raucher, Elly Teman, and Tanya Zion-Waldoks.

Many colleagues have read portions of this book, but Ayala Fader, Ben Kasstan, Risa Cromer, and Cara Rock-Singer have constantly kept me going and helped me refine my arguments so that they might be legible to other people beyond my own messy mind. Reviewers for New York University Press have helped me produce a much better book than I could have ever produced on my own. Special thanks to NYU Press editor Jennifer Hammer for being the best editor one could ever hope for. Thank you for guiding me on every step of this path with grace, patience, and divine eloquence. Nerit Zeliger assisted in the graphic design for the book cover, enriching this book with her keen eye and fine aesthetics. Thanks to Tamar Greenbaum's recommendation, Avishag Shaar-Yashuv came on board at the exact right moment, enhancing this book with her extraordinary photography. Thank you for offering such uniquely positioned visualizations for many of the themes that emerge in this book.

At the Hebrew University of Jerusalem, I want to thank my colleagues at the Department of Sociology and Anthropology, the Program in Cultural Studies, and the Federmann School of Public Policy and Governance for their fabulous support. I am especially grateful to the administrative team—Ofra, Roni, Tom, Inbal, and Maya—for their constant care. I also thank my colleagues at the Technion Institute of Technology and the University of Haifa for venturing together on new paths at the intersection of religion and science: Ayelet Baram-Tsabari, Oren Golan, Nakhi Mishol-Shauli, Yael Rozenblum, and Yariv Tsfati.

Generous institutional grants supported my fieldwork and the writing of this book, including the Presidential Grant for Outstanding Students from the Hebrew University of Jerusalem, the Shaine Center at the Hebrew University of Jerusalem, and the Jewish Studies and Human Rights Fellowship from the Israeli Democracy Institute. Special thanks are due to Yedidia Stern, Shahar Lifshitz, and Hanoch Dagan.

Some of the material in this book has appeared in earlier publications. Chapter 1 includes excerpts from an article that appeared in the *Journal of Modern Jewish Studies* in 2019. A part of chapter 2 appeared in a coauthored article in *Anthropology and Education Quarterly* in 2021; I give special thanks to Ben Kasstan for his permission to include parts of this coauthored publication in this book. Chapter 3 includes some material that appeared in *Medical Anthropology* in 2019. Chapter 4 is a heavily revised version of an article that appeared in *American Anthropologist* in 2021. Many thanks to the editors and reviewers of these publications.

Finally, I would like to express my gratitude to my family. The entire Taragin-Mann-Zeller clan have constantly supported me throughout this research. Thank you to my grandparents, Tirtza and Professor Joshua Mann, and Esther and Dr. Joshua Taragin, for the unique opportunity to grow up with deep, loving, and wise roots. Your love constantly reminds me what family is all about—this book is dedicated to you.

I am forever in debt to my parents, Mark and Adina, for their ongoing support. I can only hope to give my children the kind of love and support that you have bestowed upon me. And finally, my family, the ones who are there for me on a daily basis and know what this project really entailed. I am especially grateful to my life partner, Mordechai. We both know I could not have done this without your constant love and daily support. Thank you for dreaming with me. Thank you for enabling me to pursue dreams I did not even know I had. I am also grateful to my beautiful children, Kol David, Raz Adama, and Ilana Almaya. Thank you for choosing us as parents. Your love gives us strength every day.

# NOTES

## INTRODUCTION

1. Unless otherwise noted, all translations are my own.
2. Kanaaneh 2002.
3. As I will explain in detail later, I draw heavily on the concept of "reproductive governance," which refers to the mechanisms through which different actors use legislative controls and ethical incitements (among others) to monitor and "control reproductive behaviors and population practices" (E. Roberts and Morgan 2012, 243).
4. Israel Central Bureau of Statistics 2019. See also DellaPergola 2017.
5. See Lustenberger 2020. These particular racial categories will be fully explained in the next section.
6. For more on the history of Haredi Jews in Israel, see Zicherman and Cahaner 2012; Cahaner 2020; Cahaner and Malach 2021; Caplan and Stadler 2009; El-Or 1994, 2006; Friedman 1991; Heilman 1992; J. Katz 1986, 1998, 2022; Lehman and Siebzehner 2006; Leon 2010; Stadler 2009, 2012; Taragin-Zeller and Stadler 2022.
7. It is important to note here that there are constant struggles between different Jewish denominations, with each claiming that its version of Torah-inspired life is the most authentic. See Feldman 2022; Guzmen-Carmeli 2020.
8. Arlosoroff 2021; see also Arlosoroff 2020.
9. Zionism holds different meanings for different groups. As I will explain later, during the mid-twentieth century, various ultra-Orthodox streams publicly opposed the founding and existence of a Jewish state.
10. Since these changes, Haredi politicians pushed to transform these cutbacks.
11. *Calcalist* 2015.
12. Kravel-Tovi 2017, 38. See also Navaro 2002; Navaro et al. 2021.
13. *Calcalist* 2015.
14. Cappel and Lang 2020; Davidman 2018; Fader 2017; Newfield 2020; Roda 2020.
15. Thompson 2013. In this book, as I will explain later, I borrow the concept of "ethical choreography" from Charis Thompson and rework it to demonstrate the dynamics by which technical, scientific, gender, legal, political, financial, and theological sensitivities are coordinated to make an ethical life.
16. For more on the evolution of female education in Haredi Judaism, see Seidman 2019.

17 Franklin 1997, 2012, 2013; Ginsburg and Rapp 1995; Inhorn 1994, 2003; Paxson 2004; Strathern 1992.
18 Franklin 2013, 153.
19 Birenbaum-Carmeli 2004; Birenbaum-Carmeli et al. 2021; Hashiloni-Dolev 2007; 2018; Ivry 2009; Kanaaneh 2002; Raucher 2020; Teman 2010.
20 For reproductive justice frameworks, see Davis 2020; Ross and Solinger 2017; Smietana, Thompson, and Twine 2018; Luna and Luker 2013. For settler-colonial readings, see Merleau-Ponty, Vertommen, and Pucéat 2018; Nahman 2013; Vertommen 2016; Vertommen, Parry, and Nahman 2022. Also see Sabbagh-Khoury 2022.
21 Kanaaneh 2002.
22 Willen 2019.
23 E. Roberts and Morgan 2012, 243.
24 E. Roberts and Morgan 2012, 242.
25 Foucault 1990; Fassin 2007.
26 Briggs 2017.
27 Murphy 2017, 3.
28 Murphy 2017, 4.
29 As Yaakov Yadgar has recently put it, there is "a predominant sense of a categorical distinction between matters that are internal to Israeli sociopolitics (i.e., what we would usually call national politics), which are supposedly of only implicit relevance to this conflict, and matters that are international and bear directly on it. The internal issues—dealing, for example, with Israeli/Zionist national identity, religion, and politics in Israel, Israeli political culture, Jewish identity in Israel, etc.—were seen as only remotely and indirectly influencing the actions taken by Israel in its conflictual relations with the Palestinians and the Arab world at large. This distinction, which lies at the root of the usual framing of the discussion on a conflict that is commonly (as well as incorrectly and rather insensitively) labeled the 'Jewish-Arab' conflict, assumes the meaning of these names, or sides, to be obvious" (2020, xi). In a similar vein, I show how these "internal" categories are central to understanding state violence.
30 Bjork-James 2021; Cromer 2019, 2020, 2023; Erten and Inhorn 2020; Franklin and Ginsburg 2019; Gürtin 2012, 2016; Mehta 2018, 2020; Natividad 2018; O'Shaughnessy 2021; Saluk 2021.
31 E.g., Collins 2000; Rivkin-Fish, 2005.
32 For some exceptions, see Cromer 2020; De Zordo, Mishtal, and Anton 2016; Kasstan 2019; Tamarkin 2020; Zanini 2019.
33 Inhorn 1994.
34 For a similar move in the context of religion in America, see Wilde 2019.
35 For some exceptions, see Ivry 2009; Han 2013; Layne 2003.
36 Peri-Rotem 2016.
37 Boas et al. 2018.

38  For "quest for conception," see Inhorn 1994. Also see Seeman 2010; Weiss 2002; Sered 2000; Boyarin 2013.
39  Genesis 1:28.
40  See Irshai 2012; Kahn 2000.
41  See Irshai 2012.
42  Irshai 2012.
43  von Weisl 1941, 3.
44  Bachi 1944.
45  Davin 1978.
46  Rosenberg-Friedman 2017, 142.
47  Quoted in Rosenberg-Friedman 2017, 146
48  Quoted in Rosenberg-Friedman 2017, 164.
49  Portuguese 1998.
50  Lustenberger 2020.
51  Quoted in Birenbaum-Carmeli and Carmeli 2010, 7.
52  Birenbaum-Carmeli and Carmeli 2010, 6.
53  Batnitzky 2013. Today Jewish identity in Israel is complex, fusing different attitudes toward religion, race, ethnicity, and nationality. A study by the Pew Research Center (2016) found that Israeli Jews are divided about what "being Jewish" means. Most of the Haredi Jews responded that being Jewish is largely about being religious, while most secular Jews referred to their Judaism as a matter of cultural heritage.
54  For a recent survey of the politics of Orthodox Judaism in prewar Europe, see Mahla 2020.
55  Yadgar 2017, 13. Also see Hart 2011.
56  See Caplan 2007; Leon 2010.
57  Quoted in Rosenberg-Friedman 2017, 26.
58  Kanaaneh 2002.
59  Hashash 2004.
60  Lavie 2018, 55–56.
61  Ducker 2006.
62  Quoted in Stoler-Liss 2003, 114.
63  See Gamliel and Shifris 2019. Also see Seeman 2009.
64  Abdul Kahbeer 2016.
65  See Stadler 2009, 2012; Malchi 2021.
66  Friedman 1988; Heilman 1992.
67  Stadler 2009, 2012.
68  Friedman 1988.
69  Friedman 1988; Heilman 1992; Stadler 2009.
70  Stadler 2009, 2012; Stadler and Taragin-Zeller 2017; Taragin-Zeller 2019b.
71  For work on the complex Haredi attitude toward internet use, see Fader 2009; Golan and Stadler 2015; Golan and Mishol-Shauli 2018; Neriya-Ben Schahar 2016.

72  Katzir and Perry-Hazan 2018.
73  Frenkel and Wasserman 2020.
74  Merleau-Ponty, Vertommen, and Pucéat 2018.
75  Thompson 2005.
76  E. Roberts 2012, 7–16.
77  Franklin 1997; Inhorn 2006, 427–28
78  Bharadwaj 2016; Bharadwaj et al. 2005; Clarke 2009; Inhorn 2003; Kahn 2000; Paxson 2004.
79  While anxieties around egg and sperm donation were met with creativity by both Jewish and Muslim scholars, Catholics, Evangelicals, and Mormons were more hesitant. See Kahn 2000; Inhorn 2003; Clarke 2009.
80  Inhorn 2015, 22.
81  Inhorn 2015; Kleinman 1992; Rapp 1988.
82  For Iran, see Tremayne 2015; for Lebanon, see Clarke 2009; for Turkey, see Gürtin 2016.
83  Kanaaneh 2002.
84  Paxson 2004, 19.
85  Kahn 2000.
86  Asad 1993.
87  Asad 1993, 2003; Mahmood 2005.
88  Osella and Soares 2010, 11; Sehlikoglu 2021.
89  Fader 2020.
90  Gaddini 2021.
91  Pelkmans 2013, 1.
92  Davidman 2018; Fader 2017; Newfield 2020.
93  Cf. Deutsch and Casper 2021; Fader 2009, 2020; Stadler 2009; Tavory 2016.
94  Kasstan 2019.
95  See Mahmood 2016.
96  For example, Michal Kravel-Tovi has systematically utilized a biopolitics lens to understand how minority populations are managed. I draw on her understanding that biopolitics "constitutes a domain of practice through which the state engages with questions, anxieties, and ideals concerning its population" (2017, 31).
97  Ahmed 2006a, 2006b.
98  Ahmed 2006b, 92.
99  Candea 2018, 3. Also see Strathern 2020.
100 Mauss (1922) 1990; Douglas 1966.
101 Taragin-Zeller and Kasstan 2021.
102 For more on the particular dimensions of Hasidic Judaism, see Magid 2014; Fader 2009, 2020. For a survey of modern-Orthodox Judaism, see De Lange, Michael and Freud-Kandel 2005.
103 Kanaaneh 2002, 8.
104 Boyarin 2013; Fader 2020; Kahn 2000; Kasstan 2019.

105  For a similar discussion of this dilemma in the Christian context, see Harding 1991.
106  Colen 1995.
107  See Behar and Gordon 1995.

## CHAPTER 1. CRACKS

1. For more on religious women navigating social change on stage, see Munro 2020.
2. For a detailed account of Jewish sex education, see Taragin-Zeller and Kasstan 2021.
3. For an account of the ways this silence perpetuates modes of sexual violence and troubles notions of consent, see Fletcher 2021; and Kravel-Tovi 2020.
4. Avishai 2008b; Hartman and Marmon 2004; Schwartz, 2013. In accordance with these laws, married women self-regulate their bodies as bleeding, spotting, or other irregularities demarcate a woman as being in a *niddah*, a time when sexual intercourse or any other contact is prohibited until immersion in a *mikvah*. While purity laws have been a locus of struggles throughout generations, they have also served as a creative and concealed type of contraception (of sorts). Namely, by putting off the time of immersion, sexual relations may be delayed until the fertility window has passed.
5. Over the last thirty years there has been a rapid increase in the number of marriage guidebooks, which can be purchased in Haredi bookstores; see Novis-Deutsch and Engelberg 2012. There has also been a growth in the number of available marriage courses, which reflects how couples have to invest effort to bridge the knowledge gaps caused by an educational vacuum.
6. See Fader 2020.
7. Insurance Institute in Israel 2016.
8. Toledano et al., 2011.
9. Frenkel and Wasserman 2020; Stadler 2009; Stadler and Taragin-Zeller 2017.
10. Stadler 2009.
11. Hays 1996. Also see Faircloth 2013.
12. Golden, Erdreich, and Robermen 2018.
13. Hays 1996, x.
14. Raucher 2020.
15. El-Or 1997; Finkelman 2011; Layosh 2014.
16. Leon and Lavie 2013.
17. See Hakak 2016; Wagner 2017.
18. Ari Engelberg has documented this frustration and demonstrated how couples search for ways to create intimacy before marriage. See Engelberg 2011.
19. For a detailed account of STEM education among Haredim in Israel, see Barak-Corren and Perry-Hazan 2021; Katzir and Perry-Hazan 2018; Taragin-Zeller, Rozenblum, and Baram-Tsabari 2020, 2022.

20 Katan 2012, 53. In contrast to most names in this chapter, which are pseudonyms, Dr. Chana Katan is her real name, which I have not changed because I refer to her public views as they appear in her published books.
21 Katan 2012, 48.
22 For a detailed look at beauty and biopolitics, see Liebelt 2021.
23 Inhorn 2003.
24 Kehana 2009, 76.
25 Rabbi Joshua asserts that one must never stop procreating (BT Yevamot 62b). Some authorities interpreted this as a rabbinic (*derabanan*) determination meant to annul the limitation on the number of children needed (e.g., Rif, Baal Hamaor, Rosh) while others understood it as a suggestion (e.g., Ramban). The halachic debate about procreation also includes lengthy debates about permitted birth control methods. Today, the Pill and the IUD have become the most preferred methods of birth control; see Irshai 2012.
26 Irshai 2012.
27 E.g., Shulchan Aruch, Aruch Hashulchan Even Haezer 1:8.
28 Okun 2013.
29 Ahmed 2006a, 554.
30 Ahmed 2006a, 555.
31 Even though I am well aware that queer disorientation is up against entrenched social sanctions and stigma, here I focus on the similarities between the groups as they reorient themselves amid changing social norms.
32 Ahmed 2006a, 554.

## CHAPTER 2. REPRO-THEOLOGIES IN THE PROMISED LAND

1 Because this research project focused on contemporary discourse, the data were not collected to compare historical versus current discourses. For a historical analysis, see Rosenberg-Friedman 2017.
2 Also see Bender 2003.
3 See Kahn 2000; Irshai 2012.
4 See Raucher 2020, esp. chap. 4.
5 See Phan 2020; Furani 2019; Lemons 2018; Meneses and Bronkema 2017; Mathews and Tomlinson 2018; Napolitano 2022; Robbins 2006, 2020; Tomlinson 2020.
6 See Cannell 2006; Raucher 2020; Rock-Singer 2020a, 2020b.
7 Benjamin 2018, xv.
8 Binyan Shalem 2021.
9 Briggs 2017.
10 Organizations vary in their funding sources. Most are private organizations that charge fees for participation but also fundraise to support their operating costs. Some organizations work together with seminaries, yeshivot, and other educational institutions to share infrastructural costs. For example, the organizers of

Binyan Shalem teach at Midreshet Harova seminary and Yeshivat Eli, which they often couple up with, especially for large events.
11. *Yated* is a Haredi daily newspaper, primarily read by the Lithuanian Haredi stream in Israel.
12. Avishai and Randles 2018.
13. The Zohar (literally, "splendor") is a foundational work in the literature of mystical Jewish thought.
14. Hays 1996. Also see Faircloth 2013.
15. Paxson 2004, 482.
16. E. Ochs and Kremer-Sadlit 2007, 6.
17. Mattingly 2014. Also see Davis 2020.
18. Engelberg 2011, 431.
19. Boyarin 1989.
20. See Seeman 2009.
21. Fader 2017.
22. Inhorn 1994; Inhorn and Balen 2002.
23. For a powerful account, see Erin and Kefalas 2005.
24. Katan 2012, 10.
25. Inhorn 1994.
26. Katan 2012, 48–49.
27. Birenbaum-Carmeli 2004; Kanaaneh 2002; Hashiloni-Dolev 2018.
28. Griffith 2000.
29. Judah and Hezekiah were twins. The features of the one were developed at the end of nine months, and those of the other were developed at the beginning of the seventh month. Judith, the wife of R. Hiyya, having suffered in consequence agonizing pains of childbirth, changed her clothes [on recovery] and appeared before R. Hiyya. "'Is a woman,' she asked, 'commanded to propagate the race'?—'No,' he replied. And relying on this decision, she drank a sterilizing potion. When her action finally became known, he exclaimed, 'Would that you bore unto me only one more issue of the womb!'" (Talmud Yevamot, 65b).
30. "A man is commanded to be fertile and increase, not so a woman" (BT Yev 65b). For a detailed discussion of women's exemption from procreation, see Irshai 2012, 30–35.
31. Similarly to Dr. Chana Katan, Rabbanit Malka Puterkovsky is her real name, which I have not changed because I refer to her public views as they appear in her published writings.
32. Puterkovsky 2010.
33. Rabbi Yoel Katan published a critique of Malka Puterkovsky's book in *Besheva*, a Religious Zionist magazine, on October 7, 2014. This critical response elicited support for Puterkovsky's new book in the more liberal parts of Religious Zionism.

34 Puterkovsky 2014, 53.
35 Puterkovsky 2014, 334.
36 This sort of argumentation was introduced by Rabbi Aaron Lichtenstein in the past. See Lichtenstein 1988.
37 Puterkovsky 2010.
38 Raucher 2020.
39 For a critical analysis of this controversial anti-abortion group, see Agudat Efrat 2022.

## CHAPTER 3. CREATING AN ETHICAL LANGUAGE

1 Agrama 2010a; Clarke 2012; Fader 2020; Ivry 2010; Mahmood 2005; Napolitano 2015; Stadler 2009; Taragin-Zeller 2014, 2021.
2 Fader 2017.
3 Fader 2017, 199.
4 Clarke 2012, 107. Also see Clarke 2009.
5 Agrama 2010a.
6 Agrama 2010a, 2; see also Mahmood 2005.
7 Foucault 1997.
8 Agrama 2010a, 14. See also Laidlaw 2013.
9 Caplan and Stadler 2009; Leon 2010.
10 Hakak 2012; Heilman 1992; Stadler 2009.
11 Englander and Sagi 2013.
12 Zicherman and Cahaner 2012.
13 Research findings show how women all over the world are demanding access to religious texts and leadership roles; see Abu-Lughod 1998; El-Or 1994; Mahmood 2005; Ochs 2007; Taragin-Zeller 2014, 2015. While some have been inspired by feminism, and others by a critique of it, there have been serious advancements in female education in both ultra-Orthodox and modern-Orthodox communities. See Avishai 2008a; Caplan and Stadler 2009; Davidman 1991; El-Or 1994; Taragin-Zeller 2014. A growing number of female scholars have specialized in the field of Jewish law, creating new professions, such as Jewish Law Consultants (Yo'atzot Halacha), where modern-Orthodox women train as specialists in Jewish law. Today, its toll-free hotline and website receive thousands of questions daily from women all over the world. See Avishai 2008a; Fonrobert 2000; Raucher 2020.
14 E.g., Irshai 2012, 2014; Zion-Waldoks 2015.
15 Taragin-Zeller 2014; Taragin-Zeller and Kasstan 2021.
16 Fader 2017.
17 Ivry and Teman 2019.
18 Ivry 2010.
19 Dividing moral responsibility between medical and rabbinic experts after receiving a diagnosis of fetal anomaly has been heavily documented; see Kahn 2000; Ivry and Teman 2019.

20 Avishai 2008b; El-Or 1994.
21 As vividly demonstrated in Shimmy and Ayelet's narrative, gender influenced the ways they engaged with religious authorities, the ways they interpreted authoritative knowledge, and the ways their relationship with the rabbi evolved as life events challenged prior rulings. Yet, it is important to note that these gendered dynamics are already in the midst of change, together with the emergence of Jewish female scholars who offer religious consultations themselves, thus creating new configurations of gendered power and knowledge; see Avishai 2008b.
22 Agrama 2010a.
23 The ethnographic analysis of these variations runs contrary to the typical subdivisions customary within contemporary Judaism, intuitively attributing more authoritarian practices to the more "stringent" Haredim (ultra-Orthodox). As described earlier, Herschel, a pious Haredi yeshiva student, was happy to "shop around," while Naomi and Elad, who practiced Jewish law more selectively, fully submitted to rabbinic authority when their fetus was diagnosed with a serious anomaly. To be clear, I do not have a definitive answer to explain why some couples seek one particular type of religious authority. However, my findings indicate that patterns of engagement with religious authorities cannot be directly linked to religious affiliation or levels of piety, which is something that needs to be explored in future studies. Psychological studies have offered much attention to the ways personality types affect modes of authority, responsibility, and obedience (cf. Kelman and Hamilton 1989). Interdisciplinary collaborations might help shed light on these complex configurations of decision-making.
24 For example, Birenbaum-Carmeli 2008, 186.

## CHAPTER 4. REORIENTING DECISION-MAKING

1 See Strathern 1992; Kahn 2000.
2 Also see Raucher 2016; Seeman et al. 2016; Teman, Ivry, and Goren 2016.
3 E. Roberts 2012, 13.
4 See Thompson 2005. In her second book, *Good Science* (2013), she also used the term "ethical choreography" to describe how people speak about stem cell research. My conceptualization here draws primarily on her first book.
5 Such as Ginsburg and Rapp 1995; Luker 1975; Kanaaneh 2002.
6 Esacove 2008.
7 Krause and De Zordo 2012; Esacove 2008.
8 Paxson 2004, 312. See also Pralat 2020.
9 Esacove 2008; O'Dougherty 2008.
10 E.g., Lifflander, Gaydos, and Hogue 2007.

11. *Baal teshuva* literally means "master of repentance." This Hebrew term, which is often called "returnees" in English, refers to a worldwide phenomenon in which Jews who grew up among nonobservant families choose to lead observant lives as adults. See Lehman and Siebzehner 2006.
12. Hirsch 2008.
13. Simon 1978, 87.
14. Raucher 2020.
15. Hleihel, 2011; Okun 2013.
16. I also found the opposite, namely, that women were reluctant to tell their husbands that they were using contraception. This will be addressed in the next chapter.
17. Trust and mistrust in medicine and/or the Israeli medical health system came up a few times. In other avenues, I have studied these questions, most recently in the context of the COVID-19 pandemic. For more, see Taragin-Zeller, Rozenblum, and Baram-Tsabari 2020, 2022.
18. Raucher 2020.
19. Seeman et al. 2016.
20. Seeman et al. 2016, 29.
21. Franklin 2013; Ginsburg and Rapp 1995; Kahn 2000; Kanaaneh 2002; Strathern 1992; Weston 1991.
22. By focusing on the ways couples delineate borders between the godly and the profane, I do not intend to suggest that this sort of project exists only among communities of faith. Constructing "religious people" as a separate entity, while distinguishing and demarcating these experiences from those of "secular people," is a project that has been largely criticized (e.g., Asad 2003). On the contrary, I use my ethnographic findings to question some of the basic concepts scholars have grouped together while seeking to understand reproductive decision-making, and so point to the value of exploring reproductive choice and control outside the context of faith communities.
23. Bhabha 1994.
24. See Dow and Lamoreaux 2020; Schneider-Mayerson, 2021.
25. Dow 2016, 196.
26. Haredi perceptions of the environment are multifaceted, but as Shelhav and Kaplan found, they tend to oppose Israel's green movements, "which are perceived as being anti-Jewish, and they object to the perception of the environment as a value per se, as this leads to protecting animals or landscape at the expense of urgent human needs" (2003, 147). In recent years, there have been a few works studying environmentalism and sustainability in the Haredi context; for example, see Alkaher, Goldman, and Sagy 2018; Daudi 2019.
27. Kaneh 2021.

## CHAPTER 5. ENDING

1. Ahmed 2006b.
2. Ahmed 2006b, 179.
3. While explicit communal pressure to have children is common, I offer an additional account of social pressure that may not have been verbal but nonetheless entailed much force.
4. Colen 1995.
5. See Stadler 2009; Hakak 2012; Riesbrodt 1993; Robbins 2004; Zion-Waldoks 2015.
6. Mauss (1922) 1990; Strathern 1992.
7. For an analysis that explores links between photographs and kinship making, see Bouquet 2001.
8. *Merriam-Webster*, s.v. "desire line," accessed November 13, 2022, www.merriam-webster.com.
9. Friedman 1991; Boyarin 1989.
10. Colen 1995
11. See Inhorn 2012; McCormack 2005; Rapp 2001; Smietana, Thompson, and Twine 2018.
12. See chapter 1, note 25.
13. Robbins 2004.
14. Antoun 2001; Stadler 2009.
15. Stadler 2009, esp. chap. 6.
16. Irshai 2014.
17. Stadler 2009.
18. Hakak 2012, 2016; Stadler 2009.
19. Within Orthodox Judaism, it is not customary to go to a pool on the Sabbath. Even though the legal position of a pool is disputable, it has been a *minhag*, a tradition, not to immerse in water on the Sabbath.
20. For national divorce rates, see OECD 2020.
21. Finkelstein 2020. For more about divorce among Haredim, see Barth 2012; Barth and Ben-Ari 2014.
22. Katz 1986.
23. See Fader 2017, 2020 for an ethnographic analysis of the nexus of mental health within process of religious change. Also Illouz 2008 on the culture of self-help as a personal strategy.

## CODA

1. As this book goes to print, another political shift has occurred. On November 1 2022, after five sets of elections in four years, Benjamin Netanyahu's made a swift comeback to power. One of the surprises of these elections was the unprecedented success of the Religious Zionist party who reaped fourteen mandates, compared to eight in former elections. This success was due to an alliance of far-right parties orchestrated by Netanyahu to maximize his electoral bloc, enhancing far-right militaristic, exclusionary and anti-LGBTQ+ discourse and policy. While the

supporters of this alliance hope to strengthen their idea of the Jewish State, this transformation has been met with growing anxieties "that religious and political extremism will be entering the mainstream" (Kershner 2022). While the exact form of this coalition has yet to be finalized, the tug of war regarding education, security, politics and religion are all about reproduction. This struggle over the future face of the "Jewish state" exemplifies many of the themes this book addresses. I argue population politics will likely be at the center of these processes, albeit in unpredictable ways.

2 Gil-Ad 2021.
3 Gil-Ad, 2021.
4 The "day care decree" is still in court. As it currently stands, this policy change is scheduled to take place in 2023.
5 Halbfinger 2020.
6 Taragin-Zeller, Rozenblum, and Baram-Tsabari 2020. For a discussion of similar tensions amid COVID-19, see Barak-Corren and Perry-Hazan 2021; Shanes 2020; Shuman 2021.
7 This also leads to the importance of developing more nuanced models of inclusive science communication that take religion into account. I have began to develop such work; see Taragin-Zeller, Rozenblum, and Baram-Tsabari 2020, 2022.
8 See Stadler 2009.
9 See Sehlikoglu 2021.
10 Ahmed 2006b, 85.
11 See Davidman 2018; Fader 2020; Newfield 2020. However, Michal Raucher's work is a clear exception; see Raucher 2020.
12 Davidman 2018; Fader 2020; Newfield 2020.
13 Egorova 2018; Gin Lum 2014; Gorski and Türkmen-Dervişoğlu 2013; Meer 2017; Özyürek 2015; Tamarkin 2020.
14 Abdul Khabeer 2016.
15 See Bowen 2016; Fernando 2014.
16 Mahmood 2016, 3.
17 See the pioneering works of Marcia Inhorn (especially 2012) and Rene Almeling 2020.
18 For some recent examples, see Gammeltoft and Wahlberg 2014; Wahlberg 2018; Van de Wiel 2020.

# BIBLIOGRAPHY

Abdul Kahbeer, Su'ad. 2016. *Muslim Cool: Race, Religion, and Hip Hop in the United States*. New York: New York University Press.

Abu-Lughod, Lila. 1998. *Remaking Women: Feminism and Modernity in the Middle East*. Princeton, NJ: Princeton University Press.

Agrama, Hussein Ali. 2010a. "Ethics, Tradition, Authority: Toward an Anthropology of the Fatwa." *American Ethnologist* 37 (1): 2–18.

———. 2010b. "Secularism, Sovereignty, Indeterminacy: Is Egypt a Secular or a Religious State?" *Comparative Studies in Society and History* 52 (3): 495–523.

Agudat Efrat. 2022. Website. Accessed March 27, 2017. www.efrat.org.il.

Ahmed, Sara. 2006a. "Orientations: Toward a Queer Phenomenology." *GLQ: A Journal of Lesbian and Gay Studies* 12 (4): 543–57.

———. 2006b. *Queer Phenomenology: Orientations, Objects, Others*. Durham, NC: Duke University Press.

———. 2010. *The Promise of Happiness*. Durham, NC: Duke University Press.

Alkaher, Iris, Daphne Goldman, and Gonen Sagy. 2018. "Culturally Based Education for Sustainability—Insights from a Pioneering Ultra-Orthodox City in Israel." *Sustainability* 10:21–22.

Almeling, Rene. 2020. *GUYnecology: The Missing Science of Men's Reproductive Health*. Berkeley: University of California Press.

Ammerman, Nancy. 2005. *Pillars of Faith: American Congregations and Their Partners*. Berkeley: University of California Press.

Antoun, Richard T. 2001. *Understanding Fundamentalism: Christian, Islamic and Jewish Movements*. Lanham, MD: Rowman and Littlefield.

Arkin, Kimberly. 2013. *Rhinestones, Religion, and the Republic: Fashioning Jewishness in France*. Stanford, CA: Stanford University Press.

Arlosoroff, Meirav. 2020. "Without Haredi Integration: Israel Is Walking toward Bankruptcy." [In Hebrew.] *The Marker*. Accessed October 1, 2021. www.themarker.com.

———2021. "Elderly People Are a Problem That Cannot Be Solved. Children Are a Problem That Can Be Solved—You Can Have Less." [In Hebrew.] *The Marker*. Accessed October 1, 2021. www.themarker.com.

Asad, Talal. 1993. *Genealogies of Religion*. Baltimore, MD: John Hopkins University Press.

———. 2003. *Formations of the Secular: Christianity, Islam, Modernity*. Stanford, CA: Stanford University Press.

Avishai, Orit. 2008a. "Doing Religion in a Secular World: Women in Conservative Religions and the Question of Agency." *Gender & Society* 22 (4): 409–33.

———. 2008b. "Halakhic Niddah Consultants and the Orthodox Women's Movement in Israel." *Journal of Modern Jewish Studies* 7 (2): 195–216.

Avishai, Orit, Melanie Heath, and Jennifer Randles. 2018. "Marriage Goes to School." *Contexts* 11 (3): 34–38.

Bachi, Roberto. 1944. "Hayeludah be Yisra'el uvaYishuv vehaDerakhim le'Idudah." Central Zionist Archives J1/3717/3.

Barak-Corren, Netta, and Lotem Perry-Hazan. 2021. "Bidirectional Legal Socialization and the Boundaries of Law: The Case of Enclave Communities Compliance with COVID-19 Regulation." *Journal of Social Issues* 77 (2): 631–62.

Barth, Anat. 2012. "Tension and Duality: Characteristics and Social Construction of Divorce in the Ultra-Orthodox Community." [In Hebrew.] PhD diss., University of Haifa.

Barth, Anat, and Adital Ben-Ari. 2014. "From Wallflowers to Lonely Trees: Divorced Ultra-Orthodox Women in Israel." *Journal of Divorce and Remarriage* 55:423–40.

Batnitzky, Leora. 2013. *How Judaism Became a Religion: An Introduction to Modern Jewish Thought*. Princeton, NJ: Princeton University Press.

Behar, Ruth, and Deborah A. Gordon. 1995. *Women Writing Culture*. Berkeley: University of California Press.

Bender, Courtney. 2003. *Heaven's Kitchen: Living Religion at God's Love We Deliver*. Chicago: University of Chicago Press.

Benjamin, Mara. 2018. *The Obligated Self: Maternal Subjectivity and Jewish Thought*. Bloomington: Indiana University Press.

Berkovitch, Nitza. 1997. "Motherhood as a National Mission: The Construction of Womanhood in the Legal Discourse in Israel." *Women's Studies International Forum* 20 (5–6): 605–19.

Bhabha, Homi, K. 1994. *The Location of Culture*. London: Routledge.

Bharadwaj, Aditya. 2016. *Conceptions: Infertility and Procreative Modernity in India*. Oxford: Berghahn Books.

Bharadwaj, Aditya, Katie Featherstone, Paul Atkinson, and Adele Clarke. 2005. *Risky Relations: Family, Kinship and the New Genetics*. Oxford: Berghahn Books.

Binyan Shalem. 2021. Website. [In Hebrew.] Accessed September 1, 2021. www.binyan-shalem.org.

Birenbaum-Carmeli, Daphna. 2004. "Cheaper Than a Newcomer: On the Political Economy of IVF in Israel." *Sociology of Health and Illness* 26 (7): 897–924.

———. 2008. "Your Faith or Mine: A Pregnancy Spacing Intervention in an Ultra-Orthodox Jewish Community in Israel." *Reproductive Health Matters* 16 (32): 185–91.

Birenbaum-Carmeli, Daphna, and Yoram Carmeli. 2010. *Kin, Gene, Community: Reproductive Technologies among Jewish Israelis*. Oxford: Berghahn Books.

Birenbaum-Carmeli, Daphna, Marcia C. Inhorn, Mira D. Vale, and Pasquale Patrizio. 2021. "Cryopreserving Jewish Motherhood: Egg Freezing in Israel and the United States." *Medical Anthropology Quarterly* 35 (3): 346–63.

Bjork-James, Sophie. 2021. *The Divine Institution: White Evangelicalism's Politics of the Family*. New Brunswick, NJ: Rutgers University Press.

Boas, Hagai, Yael Hashiloni-Dolev, Nadav Davidovitch, Dani Filc, and Shai Lavi, eds. 2018. *Bioethics and Biopolitics in Israel: Socio-legal, Political and Empirical Analysis.* Cambridge: Cambridge University Press.

Bouquet, Mary. 2001. "Making Kinship, with an Old Reproductive Technology." In *Relative Values: Reconfiguring Kinship Studies*, edited by Sarah Franklin and Sarah McKinnon, 85–115. Durham, NC: Duke University Press.

Bowen, John. 2016. *On British Islam: Religion, Law, and Everyday Practice in Shari'a Councils.* Princeton, NJ: Princeton University Press.

Boyarin, Jonathan. 1989. "Voices around the Text: The Ethnography of Reading at Mesivta Tifereth Jerusalem." *Cultural Anthropology* 4 (4): 399–421.

———. 2013. *Jewish Families.* New Brunswick, NJ: Rutgers University Press.

Briggs, Laura. 2017. *How All Politics Became Reproductive Politics: From Welfare Reform to Foreclosure to Trump.* Berkeley: University of California Press.

Brown, Benjamin. 2014. "Jewish Political Theology: The Doctrine of Daat Torah." *Harvard Theological Review* 107 (3): 255–89.

Butler, Judith. 2004. *Precarious Life: The Power of Mourning and Violence.* London: Verso.

Cahaner, Lee. 2020. *Ultra-Orthodox Society on the Axis between Conservatism and Modernity.* [In Hebrew.] Jerusalem: Israel Democracy Institute.

Cahaner, Lee, and Gilad Malach. 2021. *Annual Statistical Report on Ultra-Orthodox (Haredi) Society in Israel.* [In Hebrew.] Jerusalem: Israel Democracy Institute.

*Calcalist.* 2015. "Netanyahu in 2003: Generous Child Benefits Will Make Our Economy Collapse." [In Hebrew.] Accessed September 1, 2022. calcalist.co.il

Candea, Matei. 2018. *Comparison in Anthropology: The Impossible Method.* Cambridge: Cambridge University Press.

Cannell, Fenella, ed. 2006. *The Anthropology of Christianity.* Durham, NC: Duke University Press.

Caplan, Kimmy. 2007. "Studying Haredi Mizrahim in Israel: Trends, Achievements, Challenges." *Studies in Contemporary Jewry* 22:169–89.

Caplan, Kimmy, and Nurit Stadler. 2009. *Leadership and Authority in Israeli Haredi Society.* [In Hebrew.] Tel Aviv: Hakibbutz Hameuchad and the Van Leer Institute.

Cappel, Ezra, and Jessica Lang. 2020. *Off the Derech: Leaving Orthodox Judaism.* Albany, NY: SUNY Press.

Clarke, Morgan. 2009. *Islam and New Kinship: Reproductive Technology and the Shariah in Lebanon.* Oxford: Berghahn Books.

———. 2012. "The Judge as Tragic Hero: Judicial Ethics in Lebanon's Shari'a Courts." *American Ethnologist* 39 (1): 106–21.

Coleman, Simon, and Pauline Von Hellermann. 2011. *Multi-sited Ethnography: Problems and Possibilities in the Translocation of Research Methods.* London: Routledge.

Colen, Shellee. 1995. "'Like a Mother to Them': Stratified Reproduction and West Indian Childcare Workers and Employers in New York." In *Conceiving the New World*

Order: The Global Politics of Reproduction*, edited by F. Ginsburg and R. Rapp, 78–102. Berkeley: University of California Press.
Collins, Patricia Hill. 2000. "It's All in the Family: Intersections of Gender, Race, and the Nation." In *Decentering the Center: Philosophy for a Multicultural, Postcolonial, and Feminist World*, edited by Uma Narayan and Sandra Harding, 156–67. Bloomington: Indiana University Press.
Cromer, Risa. 2019. "Racial Politics of Frozen Embryo Personhood in the US Antiabortion Movement." *Transforming Anthropology* 27 (1): 22–36.
———. 2020. "'Our Family Picture Is a Little Hint of Heaven': Race, Religion and Selective Reproduction in US 'Embryo Adoption.'" *Reproductive Biomedicine and Society Online*, 11:9–17. https://doi.org/10.1016/j.rbms.2020.08.002.
———. 2023. *Conceiving Christian America: Embryo Adoption and Reproductive Politics*. New York: New York University Press.
Czarnecki, Danielle. 2021. "'I'm Trying to Create, Not Destroy': Gendered Moralities and the Fate of IVF Embryos in Evangelical Women's Narratives." *Qualitative Sociology* 45 (1): 89–121.
Daudi, Liat. 2019. "Orthodox Women's Identities and Environmental Attitudes." [In Hebrew.] Master's thesis, Tel Aviv University.
Davidman, Lynn. 1991. *Tradition in a Rootless World: Women Turn to Orthodox Judaism*. Berkeley: University of California Press.
———. 2018. *Becoming Un-Orthodox: Stories of Ex-Hasidic Jews*. Oxford: Oxford University Press.
Davin, Anna. 1978. "Imperialism and Motherhood." *History Workshop* 5:9–65.
Davis, Dána-Ain. 2020. *Reproductive Injustice: Racism, Pregnancy, and Premature Birth*. New York: New York University Press.
De Lange, Nicholas, Robert Michael, and Miri Freud-Kandel. 2005. *Modern Judaism: An Oxford Guide*. Oxford: Oxford University Press.
DellaPergola, Sergio. 2017. "World Jewish Population, 2016." In *American Jewish Year Book*, vol. 116, edited by A. Dashefsky and I. Sheskin, 253–322. Cham: Springer. https://doi.org/10.1007/978-3-319-46122-9_17.
Deutsch, Nathanial, and Michael Casper. 2021. *A Fortress in Brooklyn: Race, Real Estate, and the Making of Hasidic Williamsburg*. New Haven, CT: Yale University Press.
De Zordo, Silvia, Joanna Mishtal, and Lorena Anton. 2016. *A Fragmented Landscape: Abortion Governance and Protest Logics in Europe*. New York: Berghahn Books.
Douglas, Mary. 1966. *Purity and Danger*. London: Routledge and Kegan Paul.
Dow, Katharine. 2016. *Making a Good Life*. Princeton, NJ: Princeton University Press.
Dow, Katie, and Janelle Lamoreaux. 2020. "Situated Kinmaking: Towards Environmental Reproductive Justice." *Environmental Humanities* 12 (2): 475–91.
Ducker, Claire Louise. 2006. *Jews, Arabs and Arab Jews: The Politics of Identity and Reproduction in Israel*. Working Paper Series No. 421. The Hague: Institute of Social Studies. The Hague.

Egorova, Yulia. 2018. *Jews and Muslims in South Asia: Reflections on Difference, Religion and Race*. Oxford: Oxford University Press.

Eichler-Levine, Jodi. 2020. *Painted Pomegranates and Needlepoint Rabbis: How Jews Craft Resilience and Create Community*. Chapel Hill: University of North Carolina Press.

El-Or, Tamar. 1994. *Educated and Ignorant: On Ultra-Orthodox Jewish Women and Their World*. Boulder, CO: Lynne Rienner.

———. 1997. "Visibility and Possibilities: Ultra-Orthodox Jewish Women between the Domestic and Public Spheres." *Women's Studies International Forum* 20 (5–6): 665–73.

———. 2006. *Reserved Seats: Religion, Gender, and Ethnicity in Contemporary Israel*. [In Hebrew.] Tel Aviv: Am Oved.

Engelberg, Ari. 2011. "Seeking a 'Pure Relationship'? Israeli Religious-Zionist Singles Looking for Love and Marriage." *Religion*, November, 431–48.

Englander, Yakir, and Avi Sagi. 2013. *The New Religious-Zionist Discourse on Body and Sexuality*. [In Hebrew.] Jerusalem: Hartman Institute.

Erin, Kathryn, and Maria Kefalas. 2005. "Unmarried with Children." *Contexts* 4 (2): 16–22.

Erten, Hatice Nilay, and Marcia Inhorn. 2020. "Medical Anthropology in an Era of Authoritarianism." *American Anthropologist* 122 (2): 388–89.

Esacove, Anne. 2008. "Making Sense of Sex: Rethinking Intentionality." *Culture, Health and Sexuality* 10 (4): 377–90.

Fader, Ayala. 2009. *Mitzvah Girls: Bringing Up the Next Generation of Hasidic Jews in Brooklyn*. Princeton, NJ: Princeton University Press.

———. 2017. "Ultra-Orthodox Jewish Interiority, the Internet, and the Crisis of Faith." *HAU: Journal of Ethnographic Theory* 7 (1): 185–206.

———. 2020. *Hidden Heretics: Jewish Doubt in the Digital Age*. Princeton, NJ: Princeton University Press.

Faircloth, Charlotte R. 2013. *Militant Lactivism? Attachment Parenting and Intensive Motherhood in the UK and France*. New York: Berghahn Books.

Fassin, Didier. 2007. "Humanitarianism as a Politics of Life." *Public Culture* 19 (3): 499–520.

Feldman, Rachel. 2022. *Messianic Zionism in the Digital Age: Jews, Noahides, and the Third Temple Imaginary*. New Brunswick, NJ: Rutgers University Press.

Fernando, Mayanthi. 2014. *The Republic Unsettled: Muslim French and the Contradictions of Secularism*. Durham, NC: Duke University Press.

Finkelman, Yoel. 2011. *Strictly Kosher Reading: Popular Literature and the Condition of Contemporary Orthodoxy*. Brighton, MA: Academic Studies Press.

Finkelstein, Ariel. 2020. "Marriage and Divorce Rates among Religious Jews in Israel." [In Hebrew.] *Ne'emanei Torah Va'Avodah*. https://toravoda.org.il.

Fishman, Sylvia. 2009. "Women's Transformations of Contemporary Jewish Life." In *Women and Judaism: New Insights and Scholarship*, edited by F. Greenspan, 182–95. New York: New York University Press.

Fletcher, Yehudis. 2021. "Why My Haredi Community Can't, and Won't, Deal with Sex Abusers." *Haaretz*, January 1. www.haaretz.com.

Fogiel-Bijaoui, Sylvia. 1999. "Families in Israel: Between Familism and Postmodernism." In *Sex, Gender, Politics: Women in Israel*, edited by D. Izraeli et al., 107–66. [In Hebrew.] Tel Aviv: Hakibbutz Hameuchad.

Fonrobert, Charlotte Elisheva. 2000. *Menstrual Purity: Rabbinic and Christian Reconstructions of Biblical Gender*. Stanford, CA: Stanford University Press.

Foucault, Michel. 1990. *The History of Sexuality*. New York: Vintage Books.

———. 1997. "On the Genealogy of Ethics: An Overview of Work in Progress." In *The Essential Works of Foucault*. Vol. 1, *Ethics: Subjectivity and Truth*, edited by Paul Rabinow, 281–301. New York: New Press.

Frank, Gillian, Bethany Moreton and Heather White. 2018. *Devotions and Desires: Histories of Sexuality and Religion in the Twentieth Century United States*. Chapel Hill: University of North Carolina Press.

Franklin, Sarah. 1997. *Embodied Progress: A Cultural Account of Assisted Conception*. London: Routledge.

———. 2012. *Five Million Miracle Babies Later: The Anthropology of IVF*. Chicago: University of Chicago Press.

———. 2013. *Biological Relatives: IVF, Stem Cells and the Future of Kinship*. Durham, NC: Duke University Press.

Franklin, Sarah, and Faye Ginsburg. 2019. "Reproductive Politics in the Age of Trump and Brexit." *Cultural Anthropology* 34 (1): 3–9. https://doi.org/10.14506/ca34.1.02.

Frenkel, Michal, and Varda Wasserman. 2020. "With God on Their Side: Gender-Religiosity Intersectionality and Women's Workforce Integration." *Gender & Society* 34 (5): 818–43.

Friedman, Menachem. 1988. "Back to the Grandmother: The New Ultra-Orthodox Woman." *Israel Studies* 1:21–26.

———. 1991. *The Haredi (Ultra-Orthodox) Society*. [In Hebrew.] Jerusalem: Jerusalem Institute for Israel Studies.

Furani, Khaled. 2019. *Redeeming Anthropology: A Theological Critique of a Modern Science*. Oxford: Oxford University Press.

Gaddini, Katie. 2019. "Between Pain and Hope: Examining Women's Marginality in the Evangelical Context." *European Journal of Women's Studies* 26 (4): 405–20.

———. 2021. *The Cost of Staying: Women in Evangelical Christianity*. New York: Columbia University Press.

Gamliel, Tova, and Noah Shifris. 2019. *Children of the Heart: New Aspects of Research on the Yemenite Children Affair*. [In Hebrew.] Tel Aviv: Resling.

Gammeltoft, Tine. 2014. *Haunting Images: A Cultural Account of Selective Reproduction in Vietnam*. Berkeley: University of California Press.

Gammeltoft, Tine, and Ayo Wahlberg. 2014. "Selective Reproductive Technologies." *Annual Review of Anthropology* 43:201–16.

Gerth, Hans, and C. Wright Mills. 1949. *From Max Weber: Essays in Sociology*. Oxford: Oxford University Press.

Gil-Ad, Hadar. 2021. "Lieberman Has Decided: The Children of Yeshiva Students Will Not Receive State Subsidies." [In Hebrew]. *Ynet*. Accessed July 8, 2021. www.ynet.co.il.

Gin Lum, Kathryn. 2014. *Damned Nation: Hell in America from the Revolution to Reconstruction*. Oxford: Oxford University Press.

Ginsburg, Faye. 1989. *Contested Lives: The Abortion Debate in an American Community*. Updated edition. Berkeley: University of California Press.

Ginsburg, Faye, and Rayna Rapp. 1991. "The Politics of Reproduction." *Annual Review of Anthropology* 20:311–43.

———. 1995. *Conceiving the New World Order: The Global Politics of Reproduction*. Berkeley: University of California Press.

Golan, Oren, and Nakhi Mishol-Shauli. 2018. "Fundamentalist Web Journalism: Walking a Fine Line Between Religious Ultra-Orthodoxy and the New Media Ethos." *European Journal of Communication* 33 (3): 304–20.

Golan, Oren, and Nurit Stadler. 2015. "Building the Sacred Community Online: The Dual Use of the Internet by Chabad." *Media, Culture and Society* 38 (1): 71–88.

Golden, Deborah, Lauren Erdreich, and Sveta Robermen. 2018. *Mothering, Education and Culture: Russian, Palestinian and Jewish Middle-Class Mothers in Israeli Society*. London: Palgrave Macmillan.

Gorski, Philip S., and Gülay Türkmen-Dervişoğlu. 2013. "Religion, Nationalism, and Violence: An Integrated Approach." *Annual Review of Sociology* 39:193–210.

Griffith, Marie. 2000. *God's Daughters: Evangelical Women and the Power of Submission*. Berkeley: University of California Press.

Gürtin, Zeynep. 2012. "Assisted Reproduction in Secular Turkey: Regulation, Rhetoric, and the Role of Religion." In *Islam and Assisted Reproductive Technologies: Sunni and Shia Perspectives*, edited by Inhorn Marcia and Tremayne Soraya, 285–311. New York: Berghahn Books.

———. 2016. "Patriarchal Pronatalism: Islam, Secularism and the Conjugal Confines of Turkey's IVF Boom." *Reproductive Biomedicine and Society Online* 2:39–42.

Guzmen-Carmeli, Shlomo. 2020. *Encounters around the Text: Ethnography of Judaisms*. [In Hebrew]. Haifa: Pardes and Haifa University Press.

Hakak, Yohai. 2012. *Young Men in Israeli Haredi Yeshiva Education: The Scholars' Enclave in Unrest*. Leiden: Brill.

———. 2016. *Haredi Masculinities between the Yeshiva, the Army, Work and Politics: The Sage, the Warrior and the Entrepreneur*. Leiden: Brill.

Halbfinger, David M. 2020. "Coronavirus in Israel: Cases Soar among Ultra-Orthodox Jews." *New York Times*, May 7, 2020. www.nytimes.com.

Hammer, Juliane. 2013. *American Muslim Women, Religious Authority, and Activism: More Than a Prayer*. Austin: University of Texas Press.

Han, Sallie. 2013. *Pregnancy in Practice: Expectation and Experience in the Contemporary United States*. New York: Berghahn Books.

Harding, Susan. 1991. "Representing Fundamentalism: The Problem of the Repugnant Cultural Other." *Social Research* 58 (2): 373–93.

Hart, Mitchell B. 2011. *Jews and Race: Writings on Identity and Difference, 1880–1940*. Waltham, MA: Brandeis University Press.

Hartman, Tova, and Naomi Marmon. 2004. "Lived Regulations, Systemic Attributions: Menstrual Separation and Ritual Immersion in the Experience of Orthodox Jewish Women." *Gender & Society* 18 (3): 389–408.

Hashash, Yali. 2004. "How Many Children Bring Happiness: Child Policies in Israel 1962–1974." [In Hebrew.] Master's thesis, University of Haifa.

Hashiloni-Dolev, Yael. 2007. *A Life (Un)Worthy of Living: Reproductive Genetics in Israel and Germany*. Dordrecht: Springer.

———. 2018. "The Effect of Jewish-Israeli Family Ideology on Policy Regarding Reproductive Technologies." In *Bioethics in Israel: Socio-legal, Political and Empirical Analysis*, edited by H. Boas, Y. Hashiloni-Dolev, N. Davidovitch, D. Filc, and S. Lavi, 119–38. Cambridge: Cambridge University Press.

Hashiloni-Dolev, Yael, Tamar Nov-Klaiman, and Aviad Raz. 2019. "Pandora's Pregnancy: NIPT, CMA and WGS—A New Era for Prenatal Genetic Testing." *Prenatal Diagnosis* 39 (10): 859–64.

Hays, Sharon. 1996. *The Cultural Contradictions of Motherhood*. New Haven, CT: Yale University Press.

Heilman, Samuel. 1992. *Defenders of the Faith: Inside Ultra-Orthodox Jewry*. New York: Schocken Books.

Hirsch, Jennifer S. 2008. "Catholics Using Contraceptives: Religion, Family Planning, and Interpretive Agency in Rural Mexico." *Studies in Family Planning* 39 (2): 93–104.

Hleihel, Ahmed. 2011. "Fertility among Jewish and Muslim Women in Israel, by Level of Religiosity, 1979–2009." [In Hebrew.] ICBS Working Paper Series 60. Jerusalem: Israel Central Bureau of Statistics.

Illouz, Eva. 2008. *Saving the Modern Soul: Therapy, Emotions, and the Culture of Self-Help*. Berkeley: University of California Press.

Imhoff, Sarah. 2017. *Masculinity and the Making of American Judaism*. Bloomington: Indiana University Press.

Inhorn, Marcia. 1994. *Quests for Conception: Gender, Infertility and Egyptian Medical Traditions*. Philadelphia: University of Pennsylvania Press.

———. 2003. *Local Babies, Global Science: Gender, Religion, and In Vitro Fertilization in Egypt*. Abingdon, Oxfordshire: Routledge.

———. 2012. *The New Arab Man: Emergent Masculinities, Technologies, and Islam in the Middle East*. Princeton, NJ: Princeton University Press.

———. 2015. "Introduction: New Reproductive Technologies in Islamic Local Moral Worlds." In *Assisted Reproductive Technologies in the Third Phase: Global Encounters* and *Emerging Moral Worlds*, edited by Kate Hampshire and Bob Simpson, 20–29. New York: Berghahn Books.

Inhorn, Marcia, Daphna Birenbaum-Carmeli, Soraya Tremayne, and Zeynep Gürtin. 2017. "Assisted Reproduction and Middle East Kinship: A Regional and Religious Comparison." *Reproductive Biomedicine and Society Online* 4:41–51.

Inhorn, Marcia, and Soraya Tremayne. 2012. *Assisted Reproductive Technologies and Islam: Sunni and Shia Perspectives*. London: Berghahn Books.

Inhorn, M. C., and F. van Balen, eds. 2002. *Infertility around the Globe: New Thinking on Childlessness, Gender, and Reproductive Technologies*. Berkeley: University of California Press.

Insurance Institute in Israel. 2016. *Statistical Report of Ultra-Orthodox Society*. [In Hebrew.] National Insurance Institute in Israel.

Irshai, Ronit. 2012. *Fertility and Jewish Law: Feminist Perspectives on Orthodox Responsa Literature*. Waltham, MA: Brandeis University Press.

———. 2014. "Public and Private Rulings in Jewish Law (Halakhah): Flexibility, Concealment and Feminist Jurisprudence." *Journal of Law Religion and the State* 3:25–50.

Israel Central Bureau of Statistics. 2019. *Statistical Abstracts of Israel*. Jerusalem: Israel Central Bureau of Statistics.

Ivry, Tsipy. 2009. *Embodying Culture: Pregnancy in Japan and Israel*. New Brunswick, NJ: Rutgers University Press.

———. 2010. "Kosher Medicine and Medicalized Halacha: An Exploration of Triadic Relations among Israeli Rabbis, Doctors, and Infertility Patients." *American Ethnologist* 37 (4): 662–80.

Ivry, Tsipy, and Elly Teman. 2019. "Shouldering Moral Responsibility: The Division of Moral Labor among Pregnant Women, Rabbis, and Doctors." *American Anthropologist* 121 (4): 857–69.

Kahn, Susan. 2000. *Reproducing Jews: A Cultural Account of Assisted Conception in Israel*. Durham, NC: Duke University Press.

Kanaaneh, Rhoda. 2002. *Birthing the Nation: Strategies of Palestinian Women in Israel*. Berkeley: University of California Press.

Kaneh, Tamar. 2021. "The War on Plastic." [In Hebrew.] *The Marker*. Accessed October 31, 2021. www.themarker.com.

Kasstan, Ben. 2019. *Making Bodies Kosher: The Politics of Reproduction among Haredi Jews in England*. Oxford: Berghahn Books.

Katan, Chana. 2012. *A Woman's Life*. [In Hebrew.] Bet-El: Bet-El Publishing.

Katz, Jacob. 1986. "Orthodoxy in Historical Perspective." In *Studies in Contemporary Jewry*, edited by Peter Medding, 3–17. Bloomington: Indiana University Press.

———. 1998. *A House Divided: Orthodoxy and Schism in Nineteenth-Century Central European Jewry*. Waltham, MA: Brandeis University Press.

———. 2022. *On the Origins of Orthodoxy*. Cambridge, MA: Shikey Press.

Katz, Ori, and Yael Hashiloni-Dolev. 2019. "(Un) Natural Grief: Novelty, Tradition and Naturalization in Israeli Discourse on Posthumous Reproduction." *Medical Anthropology Quarterly* 33 (3): 345–63.

Katzir, Shai, and Lotem Perry-Hazan. 2018. "Legitimizing Public Schooling and Innovative Education Policies in Strict Religious Communities: The Story of the New Haredi Public Education Stream in Israel." *Journal of Education Policy* 34 (2): 215–41.

Kehana, Kalman. 2009. *The Purity of the Daughter of Israel.* [In Hebrew.] Jerusalem: Feldheim Press.

Kelman, Herbert, and Lee Hamilton. 1989. *Crimes of Obedience: Toward a Social Psychology of Authority and Responsibility.* New Haven, CT: Yale University Press.

Kershner, Isabel. 2022. "Israel's Election Empowers a More Muscular Religious Zionism". *New York Times.* Accessed November 13, 2022. www.nytimes.com.

Kleinman, Arthur. 1992. "Local Worlds of Suffering: An Interpersonal Focus for Ethnographies of Illness Experience." *Qualitative Health Research* 2 (2): 127–34.

Kranson, Rachel. 2017. "From Women's Rights to Religious Freedom: The Women's League for Conservative Judaism and the Politics of Abortion, 1970–1982." In *Devotions and Desires: Histories of Sexuality and Religion in the Twentieth Century United States*, edited by Gillian Frank, Bethany Moreton, and Heather White, 170–92. Chapel Hill: University of North Carolina Press.

Krause, Elizabeth L., and Silvia De Zordo. 2012. "Introduction. Ethnography and Biopolitics: Tracing 'Rationalities' of Reproduction across the North-South Divide." *Anthropology and Medicine* 19 (2): 137–51.

Kravel-Tovi, Michal. 2012. "National Mission: Biopolitics, Non-Jewish Immigration and Jewish Conversion Policy in Contemporary Israel." *Ethnic and Racial Studies* 35 (4): 737–56.

———. 2017. *When the State Winks: The Performance of Jewish Conversion in Israel.* New York: Columbia University Press.

———. 2020. "The Specter of Dwindling Numbers: Biopolitics, Voluntarism, and the Making of Jews in the USA." *Comparative Studies in Society and History* 61 (1): 35–67.

———. 2020. "'They Must Join Us, There Is No Other Way': Haredi Activism, the Battle against Sexual Violence, and the Reworking of Rabbinic Accountability." *Nashim: A Journal of Jewish Women's Studies and Gender Issues* 37:66–86.

Kravel-Tovi, Michal, and Deborah Dash Moore. 2016. *Taking Stock: Cultures of Enumeration in Contemporary Jewish Life.* Bloomington: Indiana University Press.

Laidlaw, James. 2013. *The Subject of Virtue: An Anthropology of Ethics and Freedom.* Cambridge: Cambridge University Press.

Lavie, Smadar. 2018. *Wrapped in the Flag of Israel: Mizrahi Single Mothers and Bureaucratic Torture.* Lincoln: University of Nebraska Press.

Layne, Linda. 2003. *Motherhood Lost: A Feminist Account of Pregnancy Loss in America.* New York: Routledge.

Layosh, Bella. 2014. *Women of the Threshold: Orthodox Women in Front of Modern Change*. [In Hebrew.] Tel Aviv: Resling.

Lehman, David, and Batia Siebzehner. 2006. *Remaking Israeli Judaism: The Challenge of Shas*. Oxford: Oxford University Press.

Lemons, Derrick. 2018. *Theologically Engaged Anthropology*. Oxford: Oxford University Press.

Leon, Nissim. 2010. *Gentle Ultra-Orthodoxy: Religious Renewal in Oriental Jewry in Israel*. [In Hebrew.] Jerusalem: Ben-Tzvi Institute.

Leon, Nissim, and Aliza Lavie. 2013. "Hizuk—The Gender Track: Religious Invigoration and Women Motivators in Israel." *Contemporary Jewry* 33 (3): 193–215.

Lévi-Strauss, Claude. 1963. *Totemism*. Translated by Robert Needham. Boston: Beacon Press.

Lichtenstein, Aaron. 1988. "Family Planning and Birth Control." *Alon Shevut Lebogrey Yeshivat Har-Etzion*, 6.

Liebelt, Claudia. 2021. "From Manicurist to Aesthetic Vanguard: The Biopolitics of Beauty and the Changing Role of Beauty Service Work in Turkey." In *Palgrave Handbook of Critical Race and Gender*, edited by S. A. Tate and E. Gutiérrez-Rodríguez, 103–19. New York: Palgrave Macmillan.

Lifflander, Anne, Laura M. D. Gaydos, and Carol J, Rowland Hogue. 2007. "Circumstances of Pregnancy: Low Income Women in Georgia Describe the Difference between Planned and Unplanned Pregnancies." *Maternal and Child Health Journal* 11 (1): 81–89.

Luker, Kristin, 1975. *Taking Chances: Abortion and the Decision Not to Contracept*. Berkeley: University of California Press.

Luna, Zakiya, and Kristin Luker. 2013. "Reproductive Justice." *Annual Review of Law and Social Science* 9 (1): 327–52. https://doi.org/10.1146/annurev-lawsocsci-102612-134037.

Lustenberger, Sibylle. 2020. *Judaism in Motion: The Making of Same-Sex Parenthood in Israel*. London: Palgrave Macmillan.

Magid, Shaul. 2014. *Hasidism Incarnate: Hasidism and the Construction of Modern Judaism*. Stanford, CA: Stanford University Press.

Mahla, Daniel. 2020. *Orthodox Judaism and the Politics of Religion: From Prewar Europe to the State of Israel*. Cambridge: Cambridge University Press.

Mahmood, Saba. 2005. *Politics of Piety: The Islamic Revival and the Feminist Subject*. Princeton, NJ: Princeton University Press.

———. 2016. *Religious Difference in a Secular Age: A Minority Report*. Princeton, NJ: Princeton University Press.

Malchi, Asaf. 2021. *Cracks in the Consensus: The Challenges to the "People's Army" and the Model of Military Conscription in Israel in a Changing Social Reality*. Jerusalem: Israeli Democracy Institute.

Marsden, Magnus. 2005. *Living Islam: Muslim Religious Experience in Pakistan's North-West Frontier*. Cambridge: Cambridge University Press.

Mathews, Jeanette, and Matt Tomlinson. 2018. "Introduction: Conversations between Theology, Anthropology and History." *St. Mark's Review: A Journal of Christian Thought and Opinion* 244:1–8.

Mattingly, Cheryl. 2014. *Moral Laboratories: Family Peril and the Struggle for a Good Life*. Berkeley: University of California Press.

Mauss, Marcel. (1922) 1990. *The Gift: Forms and Functions of Exchange in Archaic Societies*. London: Routledge.

McCormack, Karen. 2005. "Stratified Reproduction and Poor Women's Resistance." *Gender & Society* 19 (5): 660–79.

Medien, Kathryn. 2021. "Israeli Settler Colonialism, 'Humanitarian Warfare,' and Sexual Violence in Palestine." *International Feminist Journal of Politics* 23 (5): 698–719.

Meer, Nasar. 2017. *Islam and Modernity: Critical Concepts in Sociology*. London: Routledge.

Mehta, Samira. 2018. "Family Planning Is a Christian Duty: Religion, Population Control, and the Pill in the 1960s." In *Devotions and Desires: Histories of Sexuality and Religion in the 20th Century United States*, edited by Gillian Frank, Bethany Moreton, and Heather White, 152–69. Chapel Hill: University of North Carolina Press.

———. 2020. "Prescribing the Diaphragm: Protestants, Jews, Catholics, and a Changing Culture of Contraception." *American Religion* 1 (2): 27–51.

Meneses, Eloise, and David Bronkema. 2017. *On Knowing Humanity: Insights from Theology for Anthropology*. London: Routledge.

Merleau-Ponty, Noémie, Sigrid Vertommen, and Michel Pucéat. 2018. "I6 Passages: On the Reproduction of a Human Embryonic Stem Cell Line from Israel to France." *New Genetics and Society* 37 (4): 338–61.

Munro, Heather L. 2020. "Navigating Change: Agency, Identity, and Embodiment in Haredi Women's Dance and Theater." *Shofar: An Interdisciplinary Journal of Jewish Studies* 38 (2): 93–124.

Murphy, Michelle. 2017. *The Economization of Life*. Durham, NC: Duke University Press.

Myers, David N. and Nomi M. Stolzenberg. 2022. *American Shtetl: The Making of Kiryas Joel, A Hasidic Village in Upstate New York*. Princeton, NJ: Princeton University Press.

Nahman, Michal. 2013. *Extractions: An Ethnography of Reproductive Tourism*. London: Palgrave Macmillan.

Napolitano, Valentina. 2015. *Migrant Hearts and the Atlantic Return: Transnationalism and the Roman Catholic Church*. New York: Fordham University Press.

———. 2022. "Young Kings: Marcus Rashford and Theopolitical Charisma." *Political Theology*, October. https://doi.org/10.1080/1462317X.2022.2133804.

Natividad, Maria Dulce. 2018. "Catholicism and Everyday Morality: Filipino Women's Narratives on Reproductive Health." *Global Public Health* 14 (1): 37–52.

Navaro, Yael. 2002. *Faces of the State: Secularism and Public Life in Turkey*. Princeton, NJ: Princeton University Press.

Navaro, Yael, Zerrin Özlem Biner, Alice von Bieberstein, and Seda Altuğ. 2021. *Reverberations: Violence across Time and Space*. Philadelphia: University of Pennsylvania Press.

Neriya-Ben Shahar, Rivka. 2016. "Negotiating Agency: Amish and Ultra-Orthodox Women's Responses to the Internet." *New Media and Society* 19:81–95.

Newfield, Schneur Zalman. 2020. *Degrees of Separation: Identity Formation While Leaving Ultra-Orthodox Judaism*. Philadelphia: Temple University Press.

Novis-Deutsch, Nurit, and Ari Engelberg. 2012. "Meaning Making under the Sacred Canopy: The Role of Orthodox Jewish Marriage Guidebooks." *Interdisciplinary Journal of Research on Religion* 8:2–31.

Ochs, Elinor, and Tamar Kremer-Sadlit. 2007. "How Postindustrial Families Talk." *Annual Review of Anthropology* 44:87–103.

Ochs, Vanessa. 2007. *Inventing Jewish Ritual*. Philadelphia: Jewish Publication Society.

O'Dougherty, Maureen. 2008. "Lia Won't: Agency in the Retrospective Pregnancy Narratives of Low-Income Brazilian Women." *Journal of Latin American and Caribbean Anthropology* 13 (2): 414–46.

OECD. 2020. Organisation for Economic Co-operation and Development. Family Database, by Country. Accessed September 1, 2022. https://stats.oecd.org.

Okun, Barbara. 2013. "Fertility and Marriage Behavior in Israel." *Demographic Research* 28 (March): 457–504.

Osella, Filippo, and Benjamin Soares. 2010. *Islam, Politics, Anthropology*. London: Royal Anthropological Institute.

O'Shaughnessy, Aideen. 2021. "Triumph and Concession? The Moral and Emotional Construction of Ireland's Campaign for Abortion Rights." *European Journal of Women's Studies* 29 (2): 233–49. https://doi.org/10.1177/13505068211040999.

Özyürek, Esra. 2015. *Being German, Becoming Muslim: Race, Religion, and Conversion in the New Europe*. Princeton, NJ: Princeton University Press.

Paxson, Heather. 2004. *Making Modern Mothers: Ethics and Family Planning in Urban Greece*. Berkeley: University of California Press.

Pelkmans, Mathjis. 2013. *Ethnographies of Doubt: Faith and Uncertainty in Contemporary Societies*. London: I. B. Tauris.

Peri-Rotem, Nitzan. 2016. "Religion and Fertility in Western Europe: Trends across Cohorts in Britain, France and the Netherlands." *European Journal of Population* 32 (2): 231–65.

Pew Research Center. 2016. "Israel's Religiously Divided Society." Accessed March 2020. www.pewresearch.org.

Phan, Peter C. (Ed.) 2020. *Christian Theology in the Age of Migration: Implications for World Christianity*. Lanham, MD: Lexington Books.

Portuguese, Jacqueline. 1998. *Fertility Policy in Israel: The Politics of Religion, Gender, and Nation*. Westport, CT: Praeger.

Prainsack, Barbara, and Yael Hashiloni-Dolev. 2009. "Religion and Nationhood: Collective Identities and the New Genetics." In *The Handbook of Genetics and Society:*

    *Mapping the New Genomic Era*, edited by Paul Atkinson, Peter Glasner, and Margaret Lock, 221–404. London: Routledge.
Pralat, Robert. 2020. "Parenthood as Intended: Reproductive Responsibility, Moral Judgements and Having Children 'by Accident.'" *Sociological Review* 68 (1): 161–76.
Puterkovsky, Malka. 2010. "The Art of Building a Family." [In Hebrew.] *Ne'emanei Torah Va'Avodah.* https://toravoda.org.il/.
———. 2014. *Following Her Halakhic Way.* [In Hebrew.] Rishon Le Zion: Yediot Books.
Rapp, Rayna. 1988. "Moral Pioneers." *Women and Health* 13 (1–2): 101–17. https://doi.org/10.1300/J013v13n01_09.
———. 2001. "Gender, Body, Biomedicine: How Some Feminist Concerns Dragged Reproduction to the Center of Social Theory." *Medical Anthropology Quarterly* 15 (4): 466–77.
Raucher, Michal. 2016. "Ethnography and Jewish Ethics: Lessons from a Case Study in Reproductive Ethics." *Journal of Religious Ethics* 44 (4): 636–58.
———. 2019. "Orthodox Female Clergy Embodying Religious Authority." *AJS Perspectives,* Fall, 48–50.
———. 2020. *Conceiving Authority: Reproductive Authority among Haredi Women.* Bloomington: Indiana University Press.
Remennick, Larissa. 2000. "Childless in the Land of Imperative Motherhood: Stigma and Coping among Infertile Israeli Women." *Sex Roles* 43 (11–12): 821–41.
Riesbrodt, Martin. 1993. *Pious Passion: The Emergence of Modern Fundamentalism in the United States and Iran.* Berkeley: University of California Press.
Rivkin-Fish, Michelle. 2005. *Women's Health in Post-Soviet Russia: The Politics of Intervention.* Bloomington: Indiana University Press.
Robbins, Joel. 2004. *Becoming Sinners: Christianity and Moral Torment in a Papua New Guinea Society.* Berkeley: University of California Press.
———. 2006. Social Thought and Commentary: Anthropology and Theology: An Awkward Relationship. *Anthropological Quarterly,* 79 (2): 285–294.
———. 2020. *Theology and the Anthropology of Christian Life.* Oxford: Oxford University Press.
Roberts, Dorothy. 1997. *Killing the Black Body: Race, Reproduction, and the Meaning of Liberty.* New York: Vintage.
Roberts, Elizabeth. 2012. *God's Laboratory: Assisted Reproduction in the Andes.* Berkeley: University of California Press.
Roberts, Elizabeth, and Lynn Morgan. 2012. "Reproductive Governance in Latin America." *Anthropology and Medicine* 19 (2): 241–54.
Rock-Singer, Cara. 2020a. "Hadassah and the Gender of Modern Jewish Thought: The Affective, Embodied Messianism of Jessie Sampter, Irma Lindheim, and Nima Adlerblum." *American Jewish History* 104 (2/3): 423–56.
———. 2020b. "Milk Sisters: Forging Sisterhood at Kohenet's Hebrew Priestess Institute." *Nashim: A Journal of Jewish Women's Studies* 37:87–114.

Roda, Jessica. 2020. "Representation, Recognition and Institutionalization of a New Community: Reflection on the Mediatization of the Ex-Ultra-Orthodox Jewish Life." In *Off the Derech: Orthodox Judaism in the Modern World*, edited by Ezra Cappell and Jessica Lang, 315–33. Albany, NY: SUNY Press.

Rosenberg-Friedman, Lilach. 2017. *Birthrate Politics in Zion: Judaism, Nationalism, and Modernity under the British Mandate*. Bloomington: Indiana University Press.

Ross, Loretta, and Rickie Solinger. 2017. *Reproductive Justice*. Berkeley: University of California Press.

Sabbagh-Khoury, Areej. 2022. "Tracing Settler Colonialism: A Genealogy of a Paradigm in the Sociology of Knowledge Production in Israel." *Politics and Society* 50 (1): 44–83.

Safrai, Zeev, and Avi Sagi. 1997. *Between Authority and Autonomy in Jewish Tradition*. [In Hebrew.] Tel Aviv: Hakibbutz Hameuchad.

Salmon, Yossef, Aviezer Ravitsky, and Adam Ferziger. 2006. *Orthodox Judaism: New Perspectives*. Magnes: Hebrew University of Jerusalem.

Saluk, Seda. 2021. "Datafied Pregnancies: Health Information Technologies and Reproductive Governance in Turkey." *Medical Anthropology Quarterly* 36 (1): 101–18.

Schielke, Samuli. 2015. *Egypt in the Future Tense: Hope, Frustration, and Ambivalence before and after 2011*. Bloomington: Indiana University Press.

Schneider-Mayerson, Matthew. 2021. "The Environmental Politics of Reproductive Choices in the Age of Climate Change." *Environmental Politics*. 10.1080/09644016.2021.1902700.

Schwartz, Shira. 2013. "Performing Jewish Sexuality: *Mikveh* Spaces in Orthodox Jewish Publics." In *Performing Religion in Public*, edited by C. M. Chambers, S. W. du Toit, and J. Edelman, 237–55. London: Palgrave Macmillan.

Seeman, Don. 2009. *One People, One Blood: Ethiopian-Israelis and the Return to Judaism*. New Brunswick, NJ: Rutgers University Press.

———. 2010. "Ethnography, Exegesis, and Jewish Ethical Reflection: The New Reproductive Technologies in Israel." In *Kin, Gene, Community: Reproductive Technologies among Jewish Israelis*, edited by Daphna Birenbaum-Carmeli and Yoram Carmeli, 340–62. Oxford: Berghahn Books.

———. 2015. "Coffee and the Moral Order: Ethiopian Jews and Pentecostals against Culture." *American Ethnologist* 42 (4): 734–48.

Seeman, Don, Iman Roushdy-Hammady, Annie Hardison-Moody, Winnifred W. Thompson, Laura M. Gaydos, and Carol J. Rowland Hogue. 2016. "Blessing Unintended Pregnancy: Religion and Women's Agency in Public Health." *Medicine Anthropology Theory* 3:29–54.

Sehlikoglu, Sertaç. 2021. *Working Out Desire: Women, Sport, and Self-Making in Istanbul*. Syracuse, NY: Syracuse University Press.

Seidman, Naomi. 2019. *A Revolution in the Name of Tradition: Sarah Schenirer and Bais Yaakov*. London: Littman Library of Jewish Civilization.

Sered, Susan. 2000. *What Makes Women Sick: Maternity, Modesty and Militarism in Israeli Society*. Waltham, MA: Brandeis University Press.

Shanes, Joshua. 2020. "'Hands Up! Don't Shoot! We Want Summer Camp!': Orthodox Jewry in the Age of COVID-19 and Black Lives Matter." *Jewish Social Studies* 26 (1): 143–55.

Shelhav, Yoseph, and Moti Kaplan. 2003. *Haredi Community and Environmental Quality*. Jerusalem: Jerusalem Institute for Policy Research.

Shuman, Sam. 2021. "Stop the Spread: Gossip, COVID-19, and the Theology of Social Life." *Religions* 12:1037. https://doi.org/10.3390/rel12121037.

Simon, Rita. 1978. *Continuity and Change: A Study of Two Ethnic Communities in Israel*. Cambridge: Cambridge University Press.

Smietana, Marcin, Charis Thompson, and F. W. Twine. 2018. "Making and Breaking Families—Reading Queer Reproductions, Stratified Reproduction and Reproductive Justice Together." *Reproductive Biomedicine and Society Online* 7:112–30. https://doi.org/10.1016/j.rbms.2018.11.001. PMCID: PMC6491795.

Stadler, Nurit. 2009. *Yeshiva Fundamentalism: Piety, Gender and Resistance in the Ultra-Orthodox World*. New York: New York University Press.

———. 2012. *A Well-Worn Tallis for a New Ceremony*. Brighton, MA: Academic Studies Press.

Stadler, Nurit, and Lea Taragin-Zeller. 2017. "Like a Snake in Paradise: Fundamentalism, Gender and Taboos in the Haredi Community." *Archives des Sciences Sociales des Religions* 177:133–56.

Stoler-Liss, Sachlav. 2003. "'Mothers Birth the Nation': The Social Construction of Zionist Motherhood in Wartime in Israeli Parents' Manuals." *Nashim: A Journal of Jewish Women's Studies and Gender Issues* 6:104–18.

Strathern, Marilyn. 1990. *The Gender of the Gift: Problems with Women and Problems with Society in Melanesia*. Berkeley: University of California Press.

———. 1992. *After Nature: English Kinship in the Late Twentieth Century*. Cambridge: Cambridge University Press.

———. 2020. *Relations: An Anthropological Account*. Durham, NC: Duke University Press.

Tamarkin, Noah. 2020. *Genetic Afterlives: Black Jewish Indigeneity in South Africa*. Durham, NC: Duke University Press.

Taragin-Zeller, Lea. 2014. "Modesty for Heaven's Sake: Authority and Creativity among Female Ultra-Orthodox Teenagers in Israel." *Nashim: A Journal of Jewish Women's Studies and Gender* 26 (Spring): 75–96.

———. 2015. "Between Modesty and Beauty: Reinterpreting Female Piety in the Israeli Haredi Community." In *Love, Marriage, and Jewish Families Today: Paradoxes of the Gender Revolution*, edited by Sylvia Fishman Barack, 308–26. Waltham, MA: Brandeis University Press.

———. 2017. "Have Six, Seven, or Even Eight Children: On the Daily Encounters between Rabbinical Authority and Personal Freedom." *Judaism, Sovereignty and Human Rights* 3:113–38.

———. 2019a. "Conceiving God's Children: Towards a Flexible Model of Reproductive Decision Making." *Medical Anthropology* 38 (4): 370–81.

———. 2019b. "Towards an Anthropology of Doubt: The Case Study of Religious Reproduction in Orthodox Judaism." *Journal of Modern Jewish Studies* 18 (1): 1–20.

———. 2021. "A Rabbi of One's Own? Navigating Religious Authority and Ethical Freedom in Everyday Judaism." *American Anthropologist* 123 (4): 833–45.

Taragin-Zeller, Lea, and Ben Kasstan. 2021. "I Didn't Know How to Be with My Husband: State-Religion Struggles over Sex Education in Israel and England." *Anthropology and Education Quarterly* 52 (1): 5–20. https://doi.org/10.17863/CAM.55715.

Taragin-Zeller, Lea, Yael Rozenblum, and Ayelet Baram-Tsabari. 2020. "Public Engagement with Science among Religious Minorities: Lessons from COVID-19." *Science Communication* 42 (5): 643–78.

———. 2022. "'We Think This Way as a Society!': Community-Level Science Literacy among Ultra-Orthodox Jews." *Public Understanding of Science* 31 (8): 1012–28.

Taragin-Zeller, Lea, and Nurit Stadler. 2022. "Religion in Contemporary Israel: Haredi Varieties." In *Routledge Handbook on Contemporary Israel*, edited by Guy Ben-Porat, 274–86. London: Routledge.

Tavory, Iddo. 2016. *Summoned: Identification and Religious Life in a Jewish Neighborhood*. Chicago: University of Chicago Press.

Teman, Elly. 2010. *Birthing a Mother: The Surrogate Body and the Pregnant Self*. Berkeley: University of California Press.

Teman, Elly, Tsipy Ivry, and Heela Goren. 2016. "Obligatory Effort [*Hishtadlut*] as an Explanatory Model: A Critique of Reproductive Choice and Control." *Culture, Medicine and Psychiatry* 40 (2): 268–88.

Thompson, Charis. 2005. *Making Parents: The Ontological Choreography of Reproductive Technologies*. Cambridge, MA: MIT Press.

———. 2013. *Good Science: The Ethical Choreography of Stem Cell Research*. Cambridge, MA: MIT Press.

Toledano, Esther, Roni Frish, Noam Zussman, and Daniel Gottlieb. 2011. "The Effect of Child Allowances on Fertility." *Israel Economic Review* 9 (1): 103–50.

Tomlinson, Matt. 2020. *God Is Samoan: Dialogues between Culture and Theology in the Pacific*. Honolulu: University of Hawai'i Press.

Tremayne, Soraya. 2015. "Gender and Reproductive Technologies in Shia Iran." In *Gender in Judaism and Islam: Common Lives, Uncommon Heritage*, edited by Firoozeh Kashani-Sabet and Beth S. Wenger, 126–50. New York: New York University Press.

Van de Wiel, Lucy. 2020. *Freezing Fertility: Oocyte Cryopreservation and the Gender Politics of Aging*. New York: New York University Press.

Vertommen, Sigrid. 2016. "Babies from Behind Bars: Stratified Assisted Reproduction in Palestine/Israel." In *Assisted Reproduction across Borders*, edited by Merete Lie and Nina Lykke, 225–36. London: Routledge. https://doi.org/10.4324/9781315561219-26.

Vertommen, S., Bronwyn Parry, and Michal Nahman. 2022. "Introduction: Global Fertility Chains and the Colonial Present of Assisted Reproductive Technologies." *Catalyst: Feminism, Theory, and Technoscience* 8 (1): 1–17.

von Weisl, Ze'ev. 1941. "Hayeludah bein haYehudim Haitah vaNemukhah Beyoter." *Hamashkif*, July 18, 3.

Wagner, Dvorah. 2017. "Concealed Parental Involvement: Haredi Fatherhood." In *Gender, Families and Transmission in Contemporary Jewish Context*, edited by Martine Gross, Sophie Nizard, and Yann Scioldo-Zurcher, 25–38. Newcastle upon Tyne: Cambridge Scholar Publishing.

Wahlberg, Ayo. 2018. *Good Quality: The Routinization of Sperm Banking in China*. Berkeley: University of California Press.

Weiss, Meira. 2002. *The Chosen Body: The Politics of the Body in Israeli Society*. Stanford, CA: Stanford University Press.

Weston, Kath. 1991. *Families We Choose: Lesbians, Gays, Kinship*. New York: Columbia University Press.

Wilde, Melissa J. 2019. *Birth Control Battles: How Race and Class Divided American Religion*. Berkeley: University of California Press.

Willen, Sarah. 2019. *Fighting for Dignity: Migrant Lives at Israel's Margins*. Philadelphia: University of Pennsylvania Press.

Yadgar, Yaakov. 2017. *Sovereign Jews: Israel, Zionism, and Judaism*. Albany, NY: SUNY Press.

———. 2020. *Israel's Jewish Identity Crisis: State and Politics in the Middle East*. Cambridge: Cambridge University Press.

Yuval-Davis, Nira. 1997. *Gender and Nation*. London: Sage.

Zanini, Giulia. 2011. "Abandoned by the State, Betrayed by the Church: Italian Experiences of Cross-Border Reproductive Care." *Reproductive BioMedicine Online* 23 (5): 565–72.

———. 2019 "Jesus Is in Favor: Catholicism and Assisted Reproduction in Italy." *Medical Anthropology: Cross-Cultural Studies in Health and Illness* 28 (4): 356–69.

Zicherman, Haim, and Lee Cahaner. 2012. *Modern Ultra-Orthodoxy: The Emergence of a Haredi Middle Class in Israel*. [In Hebrew.] Jerusalem: Israel Democracy Institute.

Zion-Waldoks, Tanya. 2015. "Politics of Devoted Resistance: Agency, Feminism, and Religion among Orthodox Agunah Activists in Israel." *Gender & Society* 29 (1): 73–97.

# INDEX

Page numbers in italics indicate Figures.

abortion, 14, 109; financial aid for, 52; limitations on, 29–30; prohibition of, 18; rabbinic authority on, 97–98; in United States, 13, 146
adoption, 111
adult education, for large families, 64–67
Agrama, Houssain Ali, 90–91, 103
Agudat Efrat, 52
Ahmed, Sara, 1, 32–33, 34, 35, 47, 61, 62–63, 122; heterosexuality and, 125; large families and, 144; Orthodox Jews and, 142–43
aid package for new mothers, 19
ART. *See* assisted reproductive technology
Asad, Talal, 30, 33
Ashkenazi Jews, 5, 21–23; birth rate of, 16; family education for, 70; as Haredi Jews, 22; in Yishuv, 22; Zionism of, 22
assisted reproductive technology (ART), 106
Avishai, Orit, 45, 72

*baalei teshuva* (returnees), 110, 114–15, 131, 133
Bachi, Roberto, 17
Bais Yaakov seminary, 9–10, 58; bridal training at, 70–72; large families at, 89
Baram-Tsabari, Ayelet, 141
Batnitzky, Leora, 20
be fruitful and multiply. *See* Commandment to procreate
Ben Gurion, David, 18

Benjamin, Mara, 66
Bennet, Naphtali, 139, 140
Bhabha, Homi, 120
Binyan Shalem, 68–70, 158n10
biogenetic research, 27
biopolitics, 13, 32, 156n96
Birenbaum-Carmeli, Daphna, 11, 20
birth control. *See* contraception
birth rate: during British Mandate, 16–17; of Palestinians, 17; in Yishuv, 22
Bourdieu, Pierre, 144
breastfeeding: as contraception, 111; work breaks for, 18
bridal training, 56; at Bais Yaakov seminary, 70–72; on contraception, 59–60; for Haredi Jews, 58; stratified reproduction and, 130–31
Briggs, Laura, 12, 68
Britain (United Kingdom), 17, 32
British Mandate, 16–17

Candea, Matei, 33
Carmeli, Yoram, 20
*chavrutot* (study partners), 83
child benefits, 19; cutbacks in, 6, 26, 49–50
childcare: Haredi Jews and, 53, 139–41; public support for, 139; Religious Zionists and, 140; reproductive governance and, 19
childless families, 17
China, one-child policy in, 12
*chuppat niddah*, 47

Clarke, Morgan, 90
Colen, Shellee, 130
Commandment to procreate: applicable to men only, 129; be fruitful and multiply (*pru urvu*), 15, 92, 95, 107; critical of, 104; limits of obligation, 86, 145
Committee on Birthrate Problems, 18, 19
condoms, 16; as nonpermissible, 60; for Orthodox Jews, 58, 111
contraception (birth control), 1–2, 14, 19; breastfeeding as, 111; critiques on, 105, 111; *derech* and, 127; ethical choreographies on, 113; family planning and, 119; feminism on, 29, 147; after first child, 129; flexible decision-making on, 109, 119; forced, for Ethiopian immigrant women, 5; halacha on, 158n25; of Haredi Jews, 10, 48–49, 138; intentionality for, 41, 113; in Israel-Palestine, 22; lack of knowledge on, 47; after large families, 115–16; legal concerns with, 16; menstruation and, 157n4; of Orthodox Jews, 30, 58–61, 111; of Palestinians, 29; private negotiations with God on, 110–11; rabbinic authority on, 92–93, 96, 104, 115–16; as taboo, 6, 10; of ultra-Orthodox Jews, 117–18; unwanted pregnancy with, 117, 124. *See also specific types*
couples therapy: for Haredi Jews, 69; on intimacy, 77–78; by marriage counselors, 72–73
COVID-19 pandemic, 66; Haredi Jews in, 140–42; medical trust/mistrust in, 162n17
critiques: on contraception, 105, 111; of ethical choreographies, 125; on family planning, 111; female education and, 160n13; of feminism, 39, 84; on large families, 75, 83; on Orthodox fertility rates, 76; of rabbinic authority, 91–92; on stratified reproduction, 128–29

Dati Jews, 6, 36, 37; divorces of, 137; rabbinic authority of, 97, 101; romance of, 77
delaying children, 10, 111, 129, 136. *See also* contraception
Demographic Campaign, 22–23
Demographic Center, 19
*derech* (path), 127, 132, 143, 145
Deri, Aryeh, 26
desire, 62–63, 126–27; reorienting desire, 61–62; state of desire, 8–9
diaphragm, 60–61; pregnancy with, 116
divorce, 69, 135–36; in OECD, 137
double-lifers, of Hasidic Jews, 31
doubt, religious, 8, 35, 145
Douglas, Mary, 33
Dow, Katie, 120
Durkheim, Émile, 144

early marriages: intimacy in, 77, 87; promotion of, 79–80
*The Economization of Life* (Murphy), 13
Engelberg, Ari, 77
environmentalism: family planning and, 120–21; Haredi Jews and, 120–21, 162n26
Erdogan, Recep Tayyip, 13
Erdreich, Lauren, 51
Esacove, Anne, 108
ethical choreographies, 106–7, 153n15; on contraception, 113; flexible decision-making in, 109, 120; with large families, 64; leaving space for, 113–18; of Orthodox Jews, 63, 121; rabbinic authority and, 107; on stem cell research, 161n4
Ethiopian immigrant women, forced contraception for, 5
ethnography, 6, 27, 38, 104, 148
Evangelical communities, 31, 82; *Roe v. Wade* and, 146

Fader, Ayala, 31, 90, 94
family-building, 44, 80; challenges of, 85–86; straightening objects in, 122; unwanted pregnancy in, 111
family education, 67–70
family planning, 28–30; contraception and, 119; critiques on, 111; economic factors in, 72; environmentalism and, 120–21; feminism on, 28–29, 108; as holy obligation, 83–87; for large families, 111; of Orthodox Jews, 100; rabbinic authority on, 99–104. *See also* abortion; contraception; delaying children
Fassin, Didier, 12
fatwa, 90–91
feminism, 11, 12, 143; on contraception, 29, 147; critiques of, 39, 84; on family planning, 28–29, 108; female education and, 160n13; on intentionality, 147; of Orthodox Jews, 7; on rabbinic authority, 92; Torah and, 132; yeshiva and, 132
fertility rate, 4; in countries of world, 36; of Haredi Jews, 26–27; in Israel, 15; of Mizrahi Jews, 23, 77; of Orthodox Jews, 76; in United States, 15
fertility treatments, 19
first anniversary, child born before, 2, 129, 133
flexible decision-making: on contraception, 109, 119; in ethical choreographies, 109, 120; intentionality in, 109, 119
Foucault, Michel, 12, 91
Franklin, Sarah, 11, 27, 118
free loan funds *(gemachs)*, 52
Friday night: dinners, 124–25; sex, 73, 74
Friedman, Menachem, 25

Gaddini, Katie, 31
gay men, surrogacy rights for, 5
*gemachs* (free loan funds), 52
gender roles, 52, 53–54; rabbinic authority and, 161n21

gender separation: intimacy and, 78; in schools, 26
Germany: birth rate in, 17; Jihad wombs in, 13. *See also* Nazi Germany
gift: birth control as a godly gift, 112–13; children as a gift, 99, 112, 125; refusing a gift, 125
Ginsburg, Faye, 11
*God's Laboratory* (Roberts), 27
Golden, Deborah, 51
good life, 61–63
Greece, family planning in, 29
Griffith, Marie, 82

halacha (Jewish law), 5, 73; on contraception, 158n25; as an ethical language, 96; rabbinic authority and, 96
Haredi Jews: anti-abortion group and, 52; Ashkenazi Jews as, 22; bridal training for, 58; childcare and, 53, 139–41; contraception of, 10, 48–49, 138; couples therapy for, 69; in COVID-19 pandemic, 140–42; demographic threat of, 4–5; divorces of, 137; enclave of, 5, 25; environmentalism and, 120–21, 162n26; fertility rate of, 26–27; as growing percentage of population, 4–5; Holocaust and, 24–25; homemaking by men, 52–53; intimacy of, 77–78; IUDs for, 116–17; Jewish identity of, 155n53; large families of, 4–5, 7, 10, 113–14; marriage counselors for, 72–73; military service and, 5–6, 26, 141–42; older daughters as "little mothers," *131*; poverty rates of, 26, 49–50; rabbinic authority of, 95–96, 100–101, 161n24; racialization of, 23; reproductive governance by, 142; schools of, 26; as stuck in past, 144–45; Talmud and, 24–25; Torah and, 26, 50, 53; in workforce, 5; yeshiva and, 5, 26, 50, 52–53, 54, 95–96, 139; Zionism and, 5–6, 22, 23–25, 26

the Haredi Problem, 5–6
Hashash, Yali, 22
Hashiloni-Dolev, Yael, 11–12
Hasidic Jews: double-lifers, 31; religious authority of, 90
Hays, Sharon, 75
health consultations, 69
healthy food: for children, 73; in pregnancy, 80, 82
heresy, 145
heroine mothers, 19
heterosexuality, 5, 9, 19, 34–35, 69, 125
*Hidden Heretics* (Fader), 31
Holocaust, 4; anti-abortion and, 52; Haredi Jews and, 24–25; large families and, 65; Orthodox Jews and, 82, 87; pronatalist policies and, 15
homemaking, 71, 72; hardships from, 80–81; Haredi Jewish men, 52–53
housing discounts, 19
ḥuppah (wedding canopy), 119

Independence Day, 6
India, Hindu-Muslim tensions in, 13
infertility, 113; repro-theology on, 80
Inhorn, Marcia, 11, 27–28
intensive parenting, 51–52, 75
intentionality: for contraception, 41, 113; feminism on, 147; in flexible decision-making, 109, 119; hierarchy in, 115
intimacy, 143; in early marriages, 77, 87; of Religious Zionists, 79; in Torah, 78–79
in vitro fertilization (IVF), 14, 27
Irshai, Ronit, 15, 59, 133
*Ish Veisha* (Man and woman) (Khnol), 58
Islam, 28, 66; religious authority in, 90; in United States, 146
Israel. *See specific topics*
Israel-Palestine: British Mandate in, 16; contraception in, 22, 29; Jewish majority in, 4

IUDs, 48, 60, 135; for Haredi Jews, 116–17; Orthodox Jews and, 111; painful experience with, 115; for Religious Zionists, 114–15; for secular Jews, 111
IVF. *See* in vitro fertilization
Ivry, Tsipy, 11, 96

Jerusalem: family education in, 67–70; large families in, 64
Jewish law. *See* halacha; *pesak*
Jewish Law Consultants, 160n13
the Jewish Question, 6
Judaism. *See specific types and topics*

Kahn, Susan, 11, 29
Kanaaneh, Rhoda, 11, 22, 28, 29, 62
Kanievsky, Chaim, 92
Kasstan, Ben, 32
Katan, Chana, 55–56, 79–81, 158n20
Katan, Yoel, 79–80, 85
Katz, Yaakov, 137
Kehana, Kalman, 58
Keshet, Rachel, 43–45
Khabeer, Su'ad Abdul, 23, 146
Khnol, Elyashiv, 58
Kleinman, Arthur, 28
Kook, Abraham Isaac, 78–79
kosher, 143; diaphragm as, 60–61; rabbinic authority and, 96, 103
Kravel-Tovi, Michal, 156n96

large families: adult education for, 64–67; at Bais Yaakov seminary, 89; contraception after, 115–16; criticism of, 83–87; critiques on, 75, 83; Demographic Campaign for, 22–23; economic factors of, 72; ethical choreographies with, 64; family planning for, 111; with female breadwinner, 123–24; good life with, 62; hardships of, 65; of Haredi Jews, 4–5, 7, 10, 113–14; health consequences of pregnancies with,

54–57, 93–94; intensive parenting in, 75; Israeli pronatalist policies for, 14–20; mothers' prizes for, 18, 19; of Orthodox Jews, 10, 137, 143; poverty rates and, 75–76; pregnancy in, 94; religious conversion over, 126, 128; repro-theology for, 66, 70–77, 87; tax benefits for, 121; Torah and, 128; of ultra-Orthodox Jews, 114; *Vatahar Vateled* on, 43–45; of Yemenites, 22; in Yishuv, 22; young marriages for, 79–80

laws of purity *(taharat hamishpacha)*, 45

Lieberman, Avigdor, 139–40

Lithuanian yeshiva-based communities, 24, 25

Litzman, Yaakov, 140

local moral worlds, 28

luxury, 71, 72

Mahmood, Saba, 30–31, 33, 146

*Making Parents* (Thompson), 106

male friendship, Torah and, 78

Man and woman *(Ish Veisha)* (Khnol), 58

Mandatory Palestine, 4

marriage: intimacy in, 77–79; for large families, 79–80; photos of wedding, 46; poverty rates in, 71–72; romance and, 53–54; sex education on, 45–47. *See also specific topics*

marriage counselors, 72–73

maternity leave, 18, 19

Mattingly, Cheryl, 76–77

Mauss, Marcel, 33

Meir, Joseph, 23

melting pot, 21

menstruation: contraception and, 157n4; laws of purity on, 45; *niddah* laws on, 49, 157n4; sexual intercourse during, 49; at time of wedding, 47

Middle East, 13, 14, 21, 28–30

mikvah, 49, 111, 124

military service, 5–6, 26, 141–42

minority groups, 19, 32, 121, 156n96

miscarriage, 104

*mitzvah: derabanan,* 84; postpone a mitzvah *(shihuy mitzvah),* 86

Mizrahi (Sephardi) Jews: Arabness of, 22; birth rate of, 16; discrimination against, 21–22; family education for, 70; fertility rate of, 23, 77; racialization of, 77; reduced fertility of, 22, 23; returnees from, 133; in Yishuv, 22

moral pioneering, 28

moral regimes, 12–13

Morgan, Lynn, 4, 12

Murphy, Michelle, 13

Mussolini, Benito, 17

Nazi Germany: birth rate in, 17. *See also* Holocaust

neglect of children, 75–76

neoliberalism, 27, 72; Orthodox Jews and, 143; religious authority and, 90–91

Netanyahu, Benjamin, 6, 26, 139; Haredim and, 6, 139; Religious Zionists and, 163n1 (Coda)

*niddah* laws, on menstruation, 49, 157n4

*The Obligated Self* (Benjamin), 66

OECD. *See* Organisation for Economic Co-operation and Development

one-child policy, in China, 12

ontological choreography, 106

Organisation for Economic Co-operation and Development (OECD), 15; divorce in, 137

Orthodox Jews, 6; contraception of, 30, 58–61, 111; ethical choreographies of, 63, 121; family education for, 67–70; family planning of, 30, 100; feminism of, 7; fertility rate of, 76; Holocaust and, 82, 87; large families of, 7, 10, 137, 143; as modern phenomenon, 137–38; neoliberalism and, 143;

Orthodox Jews (*cont.*)
older daughters as "little mothers," 131; the Pill for, 59, 60; pronatalist policies for, 23, 47, 137; rabbinic authority of, 103; religious authority of, 91–93; religious doubt of, 8; reproductive defiance of, 35; reproductive governance and, 12; repro-theology of, 88; romance of, 53–54; secular Zionism of, 8; sex education of, 45; stratified reproduction of, 130–31; study methods and tools for, 35–39; Zionism and, 8, 82, 87. *See also* Dati Jews

Palestinians, 154n29; birth rate of, 17; contraception of, 29; lowered fertility rates of, 62; violence toward, 13
Path (*derech*), 127, 132, 143, 145
patriarchy, 8, 62, 90
Paxson, Heather, 11, 29, 75, 108
*pesak* (Jewish law), 94, 100
Pharaoh, 69, 140
the Pill, 16, 48, 147; for Orthodox Jews, 59, 60; for secular Jews, 111
planned children/pregnancy, 41, 107, 108, 109
politics of life, 12
poverty rates: of Haredi Jews, 26, 49–50; large families and, 75–76; in marriage, 71–72
pregnancy: accidental, 108; with diaphragm, 116; kit for, 55; in large families, 94; after large family, 115–16; preparation for, 81–82; rabbinic authority on, 94. *See also specific topics*
pronatalist policies: hardships from, 80–81; in Israel, 11, 14–20; for Orthodox Jews, 23, 47, 137; in Turkey, 13; Zionism and, 20–21
*Pru Urvu*. *See* Commandment to procreate
psychologists, 65

Puah Institute, 69–70
The purity of the daughter of Israel (*Teharat Bat Yisrael*) Kehana), 58
Puterkovsky, Malka, 85–87, 159n31

*Queer Phenomenology* (Ahmed), 1, 122
queer theory, 9, 34, 35, 61, 62, 142–43

rabbinic authority: on abortion, 97–98; broad shoulders and, 98, 103–4; on contraception, 92–93, 104, 115–16; critiques of, 91–92; of Dati Jews, 97, 101; ethical choreographies and, 107; ethics of, 93–98; on family planning, 99–104; gender roles and, 161n21; of Haredi Jews, 95–96, 100–101, 161n24; kosher and, 96, 103; for mediation, 98–104; of Orthodox Jews, 103; on pregnancy, 94; rejection of, 95; of Religious Zionists, 94–95, 98–104
rabbi shopping, 96, 161n23
Randles, Jennifer, 72
Rapp, Rayna, 11, 28
Raucher, Michal, 11, 52, 86–87, 111, 116
relationship coaches, 65
religious authority, 66, 89–90; neoliberalism and, 90–91; of Orthodox Jews, 91–93. *See also* rabbinic authority
religious doubt, 8, 35, 145
religious institutions of higher learning. *See* yeshiva/yeshivot
Religious Zionists: childcare and, 140; intimacy of, 79; IUDs for, 114–15; Netanyahu and, 163n1 (Coda); rabbinic authority of, 94–95, 98–104. *See also* Dati Jews
reproduction. *See specific topics*
reproductive governance, 12–13, 153n3; childcare in, 19; by Haredi Jews, 142; neglect and, 76; Orthodox Jews and, 12; as repro-theology, 70

repro-theology, 66; of exhaustion, 70–77; on infertility, 80; for large families, 87; of Orthodox Jews, 88; pregnancy in, 82; reproductive governance as, 70
returnees (*baalei teshuva*), 110, 114–15, 131, 133
Roberts, Elizabeth, 12, 27, 106
*Roe v. Wade*, 146
romance, 143; of Dati Jews, 77; of Orthodox Jews, 53–54. *See also* intimacy
Rosenberg-Friedman, Lilach, 16–17

salary supplements, 18–19
science, technology, engineering, and mathematics (STEM), 26
secular Jews, 1, 50; IUDs for, 60; Jewish identity of, 155n53; the Pill for, 111
Seeman, Don, 15n38, 117
Sephardi Jews. *See* Mizrahi Jews
sex education, 19; on marriage, 45–47; of Orthodox Jews, 45
sex therapists, 65
society of learners, 25
spermicides, 60
spheres of authority, 80, 90
Stadler, Nurit, 26, 52–53, 132
STEM. *See* science, technology, engineering, and mathematics
stem cell research, 27, 161n4
straightening objects, 122, 143
Strathern, Marilyn, 11, 125
stratified reproduction, 128–34
study partners (*chavrutot*), 83
surrogacy, 14; for gay men, 5

taboo: birth control, 6, 38; verbal taboo, 96, 100, 131
*taharat hamishpacha* (laws of purity), 45
Talmud: *chavrutot* for, 83; Haredi Jews and, 24–25; as male area of study, 100; two children in, 59, 132; ultra-Orthodox Jews and, 83

tax benefits, 18, 19; for large families, 121
*Teharat Bat Yisrael* (The purity of the daughter of Israel) (Kehana), 58
Teman, Elly, 11, 94n17
Thompson, Charis, 63, 106, 153n15
time management, 71
To be fruitful. *See* Commandment to procreate
Torah: *deorayta* and *derabanan*, 84; *derech* of, 127, 143; feminism and, 132; Haredi Jews and, 26, 50, 53; intimacy in, 78–79; large families and, 128; Lithuanian yeshiva-based communities and, 24; male friendship and, 78; religious authority and, 91
*toratam umanutam* (Torah scholars with no other profession), 140
Turkey, 28; pronatalist policies in, 13
two children: as minimum requirement, 15; in Talmud, 59

ultra-Orthodox Jews: contraception of, 117–18; divorces of, 137; female education of, 160n13; intimacy of, 77; large families of, 114; stratified reproduction of, 128–29; Talmud and, 83; Zionism and, 153n9. *See also* Haredi Jews
United Kingdom (Britain), 32; birth rate in, 17
United States, 32; abortion in, 13, 146; fertility rate in, 15; Islam in, 146
unplanned children/pregnancy, 41, 107, 108, 109, 116, 117, 147
unwanted pregnancy, 107, 108, 116, 119–20, 147; with contraception, 117, 124; in family-building, 111; intentionality and, 113; IUDs for, 124

*Vatahar Vateled* (Keshet), 43–45
veganism, 82

Weber, Max, 89
wedding canopy (*ḥuppah*), 119
*A Woman's Life* (Katan, C.), 55–56
womb wars, in Mandatory Palestine, 4
work-life balance, 52, 67, 71

Yadgar, Yaakov, 20–21, 154n29
Yaner, 69, 72–73
Yemenites: Ashkenazi Jews and, 23; large families of, 22
*Yeshiva Fundamentalism* (Stadler), 52–53
yeshiva/yeshivot: afternoon breaks in, 52; feminism and, 132; Haredi Jews and, 5, 26, 50, 52–53, 54, 95–96, 139; Lithuanian communities for, 24, 25; religious authority and, 91
Yishuv, 17–18, 22

Zionism: anti-abortion and, 52; of Ashkenazi Jews, 22; Haredi Jews and, 5–6, 22, 23–25, 26; large families and, 65; Orthodox Jews and, 8, 82, 87; pronatalist policies and, 15, 20–21; ultra-Orthodox Jews and, 153n9. *See also* Religious Zionists
Zohar, 73, 74, 159n13

ABOUT THE AUTHOR

LEA TARAGIN-ZELLER is Assistant Professor in the Federmann School of Public Policy and Program in Cultural Studies at the Hebrew University of Jerusalem. She is also an affiliated researcher at the Reproductive Sociology Research Group (ReproSoc) at the University of Cambridge.

www.ingramcontent.com/pod-product-compliance
Lightning Source LLC
Chambersburg PA
CBHW020411080526
44584CB00014B/1275